PROFESSIONAL COSMETOLOGY INSTRUCTION

By JACOB J. YAHM

MILADY PUBLISHING CORPORATION
3839 WHITE PLAINS ROAD, BRONX, NEW YORK 10467

1988 Printing

© Copyright 1969
MILADY PUBLISHING CORP.
Bronx, N.Y.

Printed in United States of America
All Foreign Rights Reserved

Reproduction of the contents of this book
in whole or part by any method forbidden.

PREFACE

PURPOSE AND OBJECTIVES

Cosmetology is one of the very important training areas in the field of Vocational Education. The importance of this educational area is readily demonstrated by the fact that, each year, over 85,000 students complete courses of training in Cosmetology Schools.

The proper training of cosmetologists requires that schools set fairly stringent standards for admission and attendance and maintain high professional standards of training.

As an instructor in cosmetology you naturally will be concerned with how you can best conduct this very vital training and teaching program. This text is designed to give some suggestions which will help you to achieve this objective.

You would not have been recommended or employed to teach in this field unless the director of your school was convinced that you knew your subject and had gained experience in the practice of cosmetology. **But, these assets alone do not necessarily make you a good teacher.** There have been many cases where prominent, capable and successful cosmetologists have failed as teachers. They may have lacked the time and interest to prepare for and conduct their classes effectively, or they may have lacked the skill to obtain class response and thus help students to learn. You have an obligation, then, to give careful thought to good teaching techniques and how to get to know your students as individuals.

In accordance with the streamlined trend of modern civilization, this text is intended to meet the need for a compact presentation of the duties and responsibilities of cosmetology instructors and to serve as a training manual for teachers-in-training. The planned objectives of the text are:

1. To provide a ready reference book which tells cosmetology instructors when where and what to do and how to do it.

2. To provide a comprehensive analysis of the duties and responsibilities of cosmetology teachers, without long and unnecessary embellishment.

3. To provide a guide for the cosmetology teacher to learn quickly the fine points and techniques of teaching.

4. To provide information and instructions to teachers in simple, understandable language, without the use of confusing technical and educational terms and phrases.

5. To provide a simple and effective guide for directors or supervisors for evaluating their instructors, and instructors for evaluating themselves.

6. To provide a text to be employed in cosmetology teacher training.

The mere reading of this text will not automatically make you a good teacher. There is no quick, easy road to success; no short cut to great teaching ability. However, your success as a teacher in the field of cosmetology is dependent upon the application of much of the material and techniques presented in the following pages. As an instructor, you are encouraged to consider the principles set forth, to discuss them with others, and, above all, to apply them to your daily work in the school. Your success as a teacher of cosmetology will be measured by the depth and extent of such application.

The Author

NOTE

For purposes of this text the words "teacher" and "instructor" are used interchangeably.

For smooth presentation "teachers" may be referred to as "him" or "her" without implying that this applies only to that particular sex.

ABOUT THE AUTHOR....

Jacob J. Yahm is a graduate of the College of the City of New York, with a Bachelor of Business Administration degree and a Secondary School Teacher's Certificate.

He became a member of the Department of State of New York in 1939, and in 1948 was appointed Examination Technician in charge of all examinations conducted by the Department of State, and has served in that capacity ever since.

Nationally, Mr. Yahm played a major role in effecting the merger of the National Council of State Boards of Cosmetology and the Interstate Council of State Boards into what now is the National-Interstate Council of State Boards of Cosmetology. He was especially active in negotiations leading to the merger of the National Association of Cosmetology Schools and the All American Beauty Culture Schools Associated—now operating as the National Association of Cosmetology Schools, Inc.

Mr. Yahm's extensive beauty industry activities are further reflected in the fact that he was chairman of the Allied Cosmetology Council for three years and editor of the National-Interstate Council Bulletin for five years.

For four years he served as Executive Commissioner and Chairman for the National Accrediting Commission for Cosmetology Schools, Inc. In these positions he acquired an extensive knowledge and understanding of cosmetology schools and teaching problems.

It is from this wide and varied background and experience that he has compiled the information contained in this text.

TABLE OF CONTENTS

1 **PERSONAL CHARACTERISTICS OF A GOOD TEACHER** 1
   - Teacher-Student Relations 1
   - Professional Qualifications 4
   - Ethical Conduct 6
   - Personal Qualities of the Professional Teacher 8
   - Good Grooming — Professional Appearance 12

2 **CONDUCTING ACTIVITIES IN THE CLINIC** 13
   - Clinic Instruction 13
   - Management of Clinic and Practice Room 18
   - Maintaining Proper Records 20

3 **PLANNING AND PRESENTING THE LESSON** 23
   - Lesson Planning 23
   - Preparing the Lesson Plan 27
   - Lesson Plan Outline 28
   - Presentation of Lesson 28

4 **CONDUCTING DEMONSTRATIONS** 31
   - Preparing for the Demonstration 31
   - Performance of the Demonstration 32
   - Completion of Demonstration 34

5 **THE USE OF ORAL QUESTIONING TO MAKE TEACHING MORE EFFECTIVE** 37

| 6 | THE USE OF AUDIO-VISUAL AIDS | 43 |

Teaching and Learning Advantages to be derived from
Slides, Films, Film-Strips and Transparencies 43
Preparation for Use 44
Presentation of Films 46
Presentation of Film-Strips 47
Presentation of Slides 48
Presentation of Transparencies 50
Following the Presentation 51
Using the Chalk Board 52

7	THE USE OF EXAMINATION (TESTS) IN THE TEACHING PROGRAM	53
8	EVALUATING STUDENT PERSONALITY TRAITS	65
9	MAINTAINING CLASSROOM DISCIPLINE	69
10	DEVELOPING A SUBJECT TEACHING PROGRAM	77
11	DEVELOPING WRITTEN INSTRUCTION SHEETS	81
	CONCLUSION	85

325 TEACHING HINTS

FOR

PROFESSIONAL COSMETOLOGY INSTRUCTION

PERSONAL CHARACTERISTICS OF A GOOD TEACHER

TEACHER-STUDENT RELATIONS

Success in teaching depends upon many factors. One of them, which greatly influences success or failure, is the teacher's relations with students. Cosmetology teachers (instructors) not only must be highly trained and skilled in the practice of beauty culture, but also, must be able to develop and maintain good relations with students. The successful teacher depends upon many small things which could mean the difference between good and poor teacher-student relations.

1. **Show that you are interested in your students—Try to understand their problems.**

    A sincere interest in your students is a most important quality of a good teacher. The successful teacher clearly indicates that he is sincerely attempting to understand his students' problems and is trying to find a solution for them.

    Remembering the names of your students is important evidence of your interest in them. Every student likes to be called by his or her name. A teacher who takes advantage of this perfectly natural desire helps to create good teacher-student rapport.

2. **Be frank and honest with students—Do not side-step issues.**

    An instructor earns the respect and confidence of his students when he either answers all their questions or frankly admits that he doesn't know the answer. The teacher who tries to dodge an issue soon loses the respect of students and of fellow teachers as well. However, if questions are important only to the individual student, do not take up class-time but answer them individually, outside of the classroom situation.

The wise teacher encourages students to come to him, not only for information on the subject of cosmetology but on personal matters as well. It is important that the students realize that the teacher is making every effort to help them.

3. **Start off right—Properly introduce yourself.**

   It is of considerable importance to the teacher that the first impression on his class, which is usually the most lasting, be very favorable. The first meeting with students should be planned with particular care. Carefully and effectively introduce yourself and the phase of cosmetology you are to present. Make a good first impression and then work hard to maintain it.

4. **Do not permit your own personal problems to affect your attitude toward your students.**

   It is not fair to permit your own aches, pains, likes or dislikes to influence your judgment or actions. The students are not responsible for your not feeling well. Students soon recognize and resent unfair treatment. Teachers must be consistently reasonable and fair in their attitudes and actions.

5. **Avoid the use of sarcasm and ridicule.**

   The teacher, who also may be a highly skilled cosmetologist, could be tempted to be sarcastic or to ridicule students when they appear awkward or slow in learning. You should consider the fact that you did not become a professional cosmetologist overnight, but only after long, tedious study and effort. Sarcasm or ridicule does not encourage or stimulate students, but rather helps to create resentments and antagonisms which are deterrents to progress and learning.

6. **Learn to control your temper.**

   The teacher who "explodes" is likely to say or do things which he really doesn't mean and usually regrets in later, calmer moments. In order to maintain proper control of the class, he must first learn to control himself. "Losing one's temper is a luxury which no teacher can afford."

7. **Demonstrate good sportsmanship.**

   Students will often make an attempt to test the ability of a teacher to take a joke. They appreciate an instructor who has a good sense of humor. They highly value an instructor who is a good sport and can accept a joke in the spirit in which it is made, even if the joke is on himself.

8. **Patience is an important teaching asset.**

   It is not always easy to be calm and patients with students, especially when their questions appear unnecessary and ridiculous. Teachers must remember that not all students possess either the physical or mental capacity to learn or to acquire cosmetology skills as quickly as they would like. Patience and understanding are absolutely essential if the instructor wishes to do an effective teaching job.

9. **Maintain professional reserve.**

    While it is important that a teacher possess a good sense of humor and keep up a friendly attitude toward all students, it is also essential that he maintain a professional reserve. In order to command the respect of your students, you cannot let the bars down too far. Students will look upon you with greater regard if you maintain the professional reserve expected of your position.

10. **Avoid over-familiarity.**

    Over-familiarity with students may often create unnecessary problems. It may lead to the appearance of partiality toward some student or students at the expense of others, thus creating resentment and tension. The wise teacher will avoid becoming, or even appearing to become, over-friendly with any student.

11. **Avoid humiliating or embarrassing students.**

    Embarrassing a student before fellow-students humiliates him and tends to destroy self-respect. If you must reprimand a student, do it in private. Humiliating him before others is one of the major errors which a teacher can make. This action results in a loss of respect for the teacher and creates resentment and loss of confidence which are difficult to overcome.

12. **Praise good work of students.**

    In order to learn effectively, students must feel that they are making progress. When they feel that they are accomplishing their objectives, they are stimulated to greater efforts to continue. Be positive in your statements to students. Do not hesitate to commend them whenever they deserve it.

13. **Seek information of student reaction to your teaching.**

    Progressive teachers will discover that they can learn a great deal about their teaching effectiveness from their students, and should make every effort to obtain reactions and suggestions from them.

    Students should be encouraged to express their reactions frankly and thoroughly. If they are sure that their comments and statements will not adversely affect their own marks, students will be open and outspoken in their evaluations.

    It is surprising how much teachers can learn from these responses. When accepted in the proper spirit, these statements may be of great assistance in improving teaching and, in fact, the entire educational program.

Good teachers eagerly seek out this revealing information and the constructive suggestions contained therein.

14. **Students should be judged on present accomplishments—not on past results.**

    All students must be rated objectively on the learning and technical performance in your class. Teachers should not be influenced by past performance or reputation, whether it is good or bad. Each students starts with the same clean slate. Your evaluation must indicate the quality of performance actually witnessed by you and must not be influenced by what was done before.

PROFESSIONAL QUALIFICATIONS

A cosmetology instructor is a member of a very respected and important teaching profession. As a part of this profession, he or she assumes the responsibility of conducting himself or herself in a manner which will reflect honor and credit to all fellow teachers. The good cosmetology teacher must have a truly professional attitude which is demonstrated in all activities.

1. **Constantly try to improve your own as well as all other teaching techniques.**

    As a teacher of beauty culture you have a two-fold responsibility. First, it is your duty to your students, and to your profession, to constantly endeavor to improve your own teaching methods and techniques. Secondly, you should try to make constructive suggestions for the improvement of cosmetology training in general.

    The fact that you are directly and closely in contact with students presents the opportunity to observe their reactions and frequently helps to develop solutions to teaching and learning problems. These ideas should be passed on to fellow instructors and supervisors, who should welcome and willingly consider all suggestions made for improving their own techniques.

2. **Eagerly accept constructive criticism.**

    Your own instruction will inevitably be improved if you will gracefully and eagerly accept, and thoroughly consider, suggestions from others. They should be accepted with an open mind since they may help to solve difficult instructional problems for you.

3. **Maintain your professional training.**

    The professional training of a teacher involves constant study. New teaching methods, new ideas being presented could help to improve your own instruction. Teacher training classes and teachers' seminars should be attended for additional knowledge of teaching techniques. The cosmetology teacher should make every effort to constantly improve professionally, as a service to students and the school.

4. **Keep up with trade developments.**

   The practice of beauty culture is rapidly and constantly changing. It is essential that teachers keep up with new developments, new techniques, new equipment and new trends in beauty culture in order that their teaching techniques be kept up-to-date. It is advisable to subscribe to and read trade publications in order to obtain information on new developments.

5. **Teaching provides an opportunity to serve the cosmetology profession.**

   The future well-being of the practice of cosmetology is dependent upon a continuous supply of well-trained, new practitioners from the cosmetology schools. The teacher has the opportunity and privilege of training future cosmetologists and thus making a real contribution to the profession.

   As an instructor, you are responsible for developing the skill and knowledge of every student under your direction. Your opportunities to serve your students and your profession are limited only by your own interest, initiative, knowledge and skill.

6. **Be willing to share your knowledge with your students and fellow teachers.**

   As a sincere instructor, you should be willing and anxious to teach your students every skill and every bit of trade knowledge possible in the time available. You should not hesitate to discuss the fine points of the practice of cosmetology and teaching techniques with your fellow instructors, and to try to help them to do a more effective teaching job. It might also be wise, if you have the ability to capably express your ideas in writing, to submit articles in trade and professional journals for publications. By so doing, you not only gain personal prestige but you help others to do a more effective teaching job.

7. **Join and actively participate in professional cosmetology organizations.**

   It is the responsibility of every cosmetology teacher to join and support professional organizations in the beauty culture field. These associations help to guide the development of technical education and try to safeguard the interests of individuals engaged in cosmetology education. Teachers should actively support these groups in their own interest, as well as for the general good of all cosmetology education.

8. **Try to maintain the professional image expected by the public.**

   The public, as well as the profession, demand that you, as a teacher, conduct yourself at all times in a manner befitting your position. You are expected to actively support community projects and be a worthwhile citizen in every way. This responsibility applies more to teachers than to individuals engaged in many other vocations, since teachers deal with human products and set examples for students to follow.

9. **Be able to do the work well yourself.**

   The cosmetology teacher who tries to instruct students in how to perform a technique or beauty culture skill and cannot do the job well himself (herself) is incompetent. The quickest way to lose the respect and confidence of your student is to try to bluff and perform in an unskilled manner. You must thoroughly master each job before attempting to teach it.

10. **Completely concentrate on school responsibilities during the school day.**

It is your responsibility to utilize every minute in the classroom, practice room or clinic for the benefit of your students. You will gain the respect of both your school administrators and students by complete application to your job.

ETHICAL CONDUCT

Cosmetology teachers are responsible for their personal conduct as governed by the Teachers Code of Ethics. This unwritten code involves the morals, character, conduct and other qualities and actions of each member of the teaching profession.

1. **Spreading rumors.**

Unfounded rumors may often be dangerous and vicious. They may result in disastrous results for the originator of the rumor, the spreader of the rumor and to other individuals innocently involved. The teacher who spreads gossip or rumors acts to tear down the morale of the entire school. The efficient instructor exerts every effort to stop rumors at their source and discourages the spread of any type of information which may be harmful to others.

2. **Loyalty to your school.**

As a professional instructor you should be completely loyal and faithful to your school. You are obligated to support it because its strength and well-being is dependent upon your actions and attitudes, as well as those of the other members of the organization. The cosmetology teaching profession has no place for an instructor whose loyalty is questionable.

3. **Avoid the use of profane or obscene language.**

The use of profane or foul language by an instructor is a revelation that he (she) lacks the ability to express himself correctly and resorts to profanity to cover up his shortcomings. The good, professional teacher should set an example for students and insist that no profane or obscene language be used by them. The use of objectionable language is largely a matter of habit which should, under no circumstances, be permitted in the school.

4. **Do not seek personal favors or advantages for yourself at the expense of your colleagues.**

    The truly professional person does not attempt to make personal progress by undermining his associates. These actions are very quickly recognized by both superiors and fellow teachers and are major violations of the code of ethics.

5. **Avoid making detrimental or uncomplimentary statements about others.**

    Your fellow teachers will quickly become suspicious of you and your motives if you make uncomplimentary remarks or adversely discuss other people. The feeling is justly aroused that if you make detrimental statements about one person, you may also make them about others. It is wise to follow the adage that "If you cannot say anything good, it is better to say nothing."

6. **Follow proper protocol on official matters.**

    Definite communication channels are established in every organization in order to maintain efficiency. On occasions, you may feel that these established procedures only act to delay action and should be eliminated in your case. However, for your own protection, and in order to maintain smooth functioning of your school, it is wise to adhere to the established practices for carrying on official business. Do not create problems or antagonisms by attempting to bypass anyone in the sequence of communication channels set up by the school.

7. **Do not discuss politics or religion in the school atmosphere.**

    Politics and religion have very little or no bearing on the teaching of cosmetology. Some of your fellow teachers or students may be very sensitive in these areas. It is wise to avoid any reference to these controversial topics in any part of your school activities.

8. **Do not live today on past glories.**

    The highly trained and qualified cosmetologist does not always make a good teacher. The professional teacher is an individual who cannot only do her job well but also successfully teach others to do it. The past honors and acclaim received for personal cosmetology performances may have no bearing on your success as a teacher. The qualified teacher is judged by present educational accomplishments and not on past performance.

PERSONAL QUALITIES OF THE PROFESSIONAL TEACHER

Due to the fact that you, as a cosmetology teacher, are in constant personal contact with students and fellow teachers, it is important that you have exemplary personal qualities.

Even more important than knowing how to recognize and handle problems with students, it is your ability as an instructor to "know yourself." You, not your students, may be the real problem standing in the way of effective class participation and learning. You, too, may be a "type" to your students.

a) Are you a **wanderer** who rambles off on by-paths, telling of personal experiences in great detail and frequently repeat yourself?

b) Are you an **echo** who repeats, verbatum, what is in the text rather than use it as a point from which to develop your subject matter?

c) Are you a **reader** who reads lengthy passages from a book rather than converse with your class?

d) Are you a **comedian** who tells lots of funny stories and keeps the class in stitches; who entertains but doesn't teach?

e) Are you a **machine,** lacking in human interest, who displays no interest in the individuals in your class and their differences?

It's easy to see the faults of others but difficult to see your own. You, the teacher, must try to see yourself as others see you. What do you do, or say, that detracts from your effectiveness? Do you understand what your students are thinking and why they are reacting as they do? If your class is not responding as you would like it to, remember it has been said that "If the learner has not learned, the teacher has not taught."

1. **Be honest.**

    A cosmetology teacher has access to a great deal of valuable implements, equipment and supplies, and may even be required to collect clinic fees. The instructor must take every precaution to prevent even the slightest suspicion to develop that he or she is not strictly honest. Accurate records must be maintained of all funds, equipment and supplies.

2. **Maintain good poise.**

    When an instructor feels ill at ease, this uneasiness is quickly transmitted to students and fellow instructors. Self-consciousness, stammering or faltering speech, and poor physical poise are weaknesses which result in a decrease in teaching efficiency. Constant effort and practice will help develop good poise.

3. **Be self-reliant.**

    The professional teacher is qualified to solve most problems with a minimum of assistance from superiors. He does not look for others to carry out his responsibilities or perform his duties.

4. **Develop initiative.**

   As a cosmetology teacher you should show your initiative and start things humming without delay. Develop and try new ideas without aid or prodding by supervisors. Seek weaknesses in the teaching program and in your own instruction and strive to correct them. Take the lead in school activities and show students and faculty your interest and initiative.

5. **Maintain enthusiasm.**

   Enthusiasm is contagious; it spreads rapidly from teacher to students. The teacher who works with vigor and enthusiasm soon sets the pace for students who react to this enthusiasm with the same spirit.

6. **Show your resourcefulness.**

   Cosmetology teachers are often required to handle classes with only a minimum amount of equipment, implements or teaching aids. The resourceful teacher will try to acquire ample equipment in advance. You can help your class and yourself by requesting literature, charts, posters, displays, samples and other aids from manufacturers. You can also display your resourcefulness by designing and building mock-ups, cutaways, models and other visual aids and making the most efficient use of all instructional material available.

7. **Be friendly with students.**

   The cosmetology instructor who maintains a friendly attitude has the greatest opportunity for service. Students may often be required to make major adjustments. If as a teacher, you show a friendly interest in them, your students will bring their problems to you. This attitude on your part will result in a show of greater respect for you and a more favorable response to your instruction.

8. **Be tactful.**

   As an instructor you must be prepared to cope with many difficult problems and situations. You will be required to give opinions and decide upon the proper course of action to pursue without offending and you must, under no condition, show favoritism or prejudice of any kind.

9. **Be sincere.**

   Your students will soon discover whether you are sincerely interested in teaching them or are primarily interested in your pay check. You cannot hope to arouse and hold the interest or attention of your students unless you demonstrate that you are sincerely interested in their welfare.

10. **Be courteous.**

    In order to expect courtesy while you teach, you, yourself, must be courteous. You must always demand and expect courtesy from your students and reciprocate by being courteous yourself.

11. **Maintain your physical and mental fitness.**

    You are of no value to your school or to your students if you are home on sick leave. Progress in learning is often halted when classes are under the direction of substitute teachers. Teaching is an extremely difficult vocation, keeping teachers under mental and physical strain. In order to perform properly, you must maintain yourself in excellent physical condition.

12. **Cooperate willingly.**

    The efficiency of a cosmetology educational institution is dependent upon the cooperation of its instructors. The good professional teacher gets along well with fellow teachers and administrators, offers to cooperate willing in every endeavor, without reservations and consistently does more than his share of the work.

13. **Avoid distracting mannerism and gestures.**

    Any kind of peculiar mannerisms are distracting to students. A cosmetology instructor must make a conscious effort to eliminate any actions which tend to distract from the teaching and learning situation. Sometimes, a little showmanship will help to drive home a certain point. However, the excessive use of gestures may detract from, rather than add to, the effectiveness of the teacher's presentation. Distracting speech habits, such as unnecessary repetition, excessive use of certain phrases and mispronunciations also serve to distract and annoy students.

14. **Do not shout, but make sure that all students can hear you.**

    The quality of an instructor's voice may influence the success of his entire teaching program. A harsh voice, or one pitched too high, may be a constant irritant to students. The quickest way for an instructor to completely destroy the interest and attention of his class is to speak in a constant monotone. Words must be correctly and distinctly pronounced and enunciated in order that they be clearly heard and understood.

15. **Teacher punctuality.**

    All cosmetology training is organized on a tight schedule. Teaching and learning time is very important in the school of beauty culture. You should make certain that every session is started promptly and classes dismissed on time, to avoid annoyance to other instructors and to make full use of the time available to you.

    The good professional teacher never delays the starting of a class nor wastes the time of students because of his own tardiness. Common courtesy requires that appointments be kept on time.

16. **Submit accurate reports and examination records.**

    Reports and school records are completely worthless unless they are accurate and complete. You should always make a double-check of all records in order to completely eliminate the possibility of error. Late reports decrease the efficiency of the school and indicate laxity on the part of the instructor. It is most desirable that you meet all deadlines promptly.

17. **Be familiar with, and live up to, all school rules and regulations.**

    One of your first responsibilities as an instructor is to become thoroughly familiar with your school's rules, regulations, policies, aims and objectives. Your next responsibility is to interpret them to your students and see that they are carried out.

18. **Keep breath sweet and clean.**

    Offensive breath, caused by excessive smoking, bad teeth, stomach trouble or nervous disorders, is a serious handicap to an instructor. Remember that you, as a teacher, will be in constant close association with students and other individuals in the school. The associations may be adversely affected by bad breath. It is advisable that you constantly check to make sure that your breath is not offensive.

19. **Keep body clean and odorless.**

    There is no excuse for an offensive body odor. Daily shower or bath and by using an underarm deodorant acts effectively to eliminate this factor which will otherwise cause both fellow teachers and students to avoid being in the presence of an offending teacher. It is advisable to have clothes laundered, or cleaned regularly to insure freedom from odor.

GOOD GROOMING—PROFESSIONAL APPEARANCE

It is possible that some cosmetologists overlook the importance of maintaining the appearance of good grooming at all times. After years of working in the salon, undergoing periods of great stress and work pressure, they begin to neglect their own personal appearance. However, as an instructor, the situation changes, and personal appearance takes on new importance and significance.

Cosmetology schools are in the business of training students to practice, sell and promote "beauty" and "good grooming." Every instructor not only must teach the facts and techniques of beauty culture but must at all times be an example for students to follow and to emulate.

The following is a check-list for maintaining a good personal appearance:

FEMALE INSTRUCTORS

1. Take a daily shower or bath and use an underarm deodorant.
2. Clean and brush teeth regularly. Use mouth wash to sweeten breath. Keep teeth in good condition.
3. Kep the hair clean and lustrous. Wear an attractive and practical hairstyle at all times.
4. Wear clothes that are clean and neat; change and vary clothing as often as possible. Wear fresh underclothes.
5. Wear appropriate make-up to match your skin tones. Have well-shaped eyebrows and lips.
6. Keep your hands clean and smooth and your nails well-manicured.
7. You may wear a wrist watch. Avoid gaudy jewelry.
8. Wear well-fitted, sensibly styled shoes. Keep the shoes polished and the heels straight. Wear fresh hose daily. Watch out for wrinkles.
9. Do not smoke or chew gum in class.
10. Maintain a good standing, walking and sitting posture at all times.

MALE INSTRUCTORS

In addition to most of the above check-list, male instructors should:

1. Shave every day. If mustache is worn, must be neatly trimmed.
2. Dress his hair neatly or wear an appropriate hairstyle. At no time permit his hair to look shaggy and/or unkempt.
3. Wear well-fitted and polished shoes. Wear fresh socks daily.

2

CONDUCTING ACTIVITIES IN THE CLINIC

CLINIC INSTRUCTION

Clinic practice is a very essential element in the Cosmetology teaching and learning pattern. It is, therefore, of primary importance that the teacher conduct and manage all clinic activities in a most efficient manner. Cosmetology students develop their technical skills and manual dexterity by actually performing the services required in the salon.

1. **Clinic practice must conform with over-all objectives.**

    After the aims and objectives of the training program have been established, all student clinic activities should be directed toward meeting these objectives. Each student's clinic activities must be selected to be certain that he or she (the student) receives sufficient actual practice in the planned techniques.

2. **Clinic activities must be productive in the learning pattern.**

    Each student's activity must be part of the over-all design. No student should be kept overly long on any single type of service. Clinic and practice room work must be varied to cover every cosmetology skill and technique. All students should be given equal opportunities to obtain the necessary practice. Activities should be so planned that no student is ever without some constructive performance project. Clinic or practice room activities should not be "time killers" but must be important learning projects.

3. **Student cooperation in the clinic.**

    Students should learn very quickly that they cannot "live on an island." One of the important objectives of any course is to provide experience in working with others. The practice of cosmetology should be a cooperative effort. Few people in the profession work alone at all times. It is, therefore, important that provision should be made for developing a cooperative attitude on the part of all students. They must learn to work together; acting as each other's models in the practice room is one method of developing this attitude.

4. **Provide for individual differences in students.**

   Provision for individual differences is fundamental to good cosmetology teaching. All members of a class do not have the same abilities, nor do they learn or perform at the same rate of speed. One class usually has its share of slow, average and fast students. Clinic and practice room duties and projects must be designed to challenge the ability of each student.

5. **Practice room tasks must be planned on an increasing scale of difficulty.**

   In planning practice room projects, tasks should be so arranged that the easiest jobs come first. A great deal of student discouragement and frustration can be avoided if students proceed to difficult tasks after having successfully completed easier ones. Students may become disheartened if they try to perform difficult tasks without a series of successfully completed projects behind them.

6. **Adhere to approved methods and techniques; however, you must use initiative and try to improve.**

   As an instructor, you must see that all techniques are performed in accordance with accepted professional methods. However, avoid becoming dull and stereotyped in your training. Use your initiative. Look for new and improved methods for performance of techniques. Make your students feel that you are trying to teach them the latest and best methods.

7. **Demonstrate complete mastery and skill in performance of the techniques you are teaching.**

   You must be able to do the job yourself, and do it well. If you do not have complete control of each technique or job, develop the required professional skill by practice or study. In order to be a competent teacher, you must be able to perform well yourself before you can teach others.

8. **Set a good example for students to follow.**

   A teacher's attitude is contagious.

   If you show a feeling of antagonism for your school, or indicate that you do not like the conditions prevailing, your attitudes may soon be transferred to your students and reflect in a lowering of their morale.

   Show real drive and enthusiasm in your classroom activities, this will be reflected in the enthusiasm and eagerness of your class. Conversely a lackadaisical approach by the teacher will result in a lackadaisical class.

Leadership can be learned from a good leader. Demonstrate and practice the qualities of good leadership in order that you may guide your class toward the development of these qualities.

Cooperation can be taught by demonstrating cooperation. Show that you wholeheartedly cooperate with the school's administration, fellow teachers and students.

9. **Develop and sustain interest by relating student activities to professional cosmetology practice.**

    Students are usually restless and curious. They like to know why they are required to do certain things in the practice room. Point out the reason for each operation and explain how it relates to the practice of cosmetology in the salon.

10. **Be alert and guard against students developing poor work habits.**

    Work habits formed in the school are carried over into salon practice. "Practice does not make perfect—only perfect practice makes for perfection."

    Techniques and skills incorrectly learned must be unlearned. Retraining is more difficult than original training, since bad work habits must be destroyed and new, correct ones developed. Watch all procedures carefully and insist that correct, professional methods be followed.

    Your supervision must be thorough and careful at all times and especially so when a new skill or technique is presented.

11. **Never do the job for students. but guide, direct and ask questions which lead to correct solutions.**

    Students learn physical and manual skills best by doing the jobs themselves. When students cannot perform properly, you, as the instructor, should guide them and ask them questions which direct their thinking toward solutions of the problems. You may even repeat part of any demonstration given earlier in order to clarify the work. However, in the final analysis the students must do their own work and their own thinking, if they are to learn. Therefore, you must not actually perform students' tasks for them.

12. **When criticizing student's practical work, always explain why its does not meet professional standards and explain how it can be improved.**

    Be constructive in your criticism. Every student effort in the practice room or clinic has some good points. Therefore, in order to maintain student interest and enthusiasm, it is best to compliment and discuss these points first. Then you may proceed to constructively criticize and point out areas needing improvement and explain how they can be improved. Make your student part of the criticizing team by asking questions such as "how do you think this work can be improved?", etc., to stimulate thinking.

13. **Instruction should be continuous.**

    Students learn better when they are under constant supervision. A teacher cannot depend upon demonstrations, lectures or instruction sheets to do the complete job of teaching. Competent, professional cosmetology teachers constantly check and correct procedures and techniques, quality of work, use of equipment and implements, application of all types of cosmetics and supplies, use of safety precautions and strictly observe sanitary measures while performing cosmetology services.

14. **Give praise to students for outstanding work or effort.**

    It isn't enough just to criticize poor work or to tell students when they are wrong. More progress is made in the field of education through commendation rather than condemnation. When a student performs well, does good work or makes a real effort to do the job, he or she should be commended. An occasional pat on the back for deserving students is good teaching procedure. Students look for deserved praise and when given, adds to more student effort, creates greater interest, and maintains or increases learning incentive.

15. **Watch for student fatigue and act immediately when observed.**

    When practice room work is difficult or monotonous, watch carefully for any signs of student fatigue. Interest and incentive begin to lag and accident hazard increases in proportion to the tiredness present.

    It is good teaching procedure to correct a condition adding to student fatigue by varying student activities and methods of instruction.

16. **Provide for special attention and assistance for slower students with learning difficulties.**

    The progress of an entire group should not be impaired because a few students are finding it difficult to absorb the material or develop proper skills. The faster students should first be assigned to their practice or training projects; then special consideration should be given to the slower students. They should be taken as a separate group and given further instruction and guidance.

17. **Use visual aids to demonstrate professional techniques.**

    Practice room equipment should be supplemented by the wise use of visual aids in the teaching program. As a rule, while most cosmetology techniques can actually be demonstrated and practiced on either mannequins or live models, a complete picture can more readily be developed by the use of visual aids. The proper use of films, charts, film strips, slides, etc. can be of great value in the teaching-learning program.

18. **Display work and accomplishment charts to develop competitive spirit, as teaching and learning aids.**

    Most students have an inborn competitive spirit. You should learn to capitalize on this. Select good work and display it as an example for other students.

It is advantageous to periodically post the amount and quality of practice work performed by all students. The students themselves can then make their own comparisons and allow their natural competitive spirits to react.

19. **Emphasize safety precautions.**

One very important area in cosmetology instruction is to teach safety precautions with every technique taught. You must then insist that all such safety precautions be followed to the letter. You must serve as a constant example by practicing safety rules yourself. Students cannot be expected to observe these rules if the instructor does not pay attention to them.

Stress the hazards involved in the use of all cosmetology implements and supplies. Discuss the usual causes for accidents in the beauty salon. Emphasize that care and alertness reduce the possibility of accidents. Point out the health hazards which may be present in the use of certain chemicals and teach all students how to minimize the possibility of accident occurence.

Discuss what should be done when accidents do occur—whom to call, the location of the first aid kit, and the action to be taken to decrease or minimize damage while awaiting help.

20. **Limit size of class in accordance with good educational standards.**

Although class size is primarily an administrative problem, teachers should be able to voice an opinion in the interests of good teaching. Instructors should not be placed in the position of trying to teach classes which are too large to manage and where insufficient equipment, space and supplies are available.

21. **Have reference material available for students.**

Alert, progressive students often are not satisfied with the basic instructions being presented to the entire group. They may be keenly interested in, and would like to delve more deeply into, the subject matter. You, as a teacher, should have such material available and easily accessible at all times.

22. **Arrange field trips.**

Try to arrange field trips to active salons in your area. Such trips will permit your students to absorb the actual salon atmosphere, to observe work and techniques employed by professional cosmetologists and to associate their own school work with actual salon practice.

MANAGEMENT OF CLINIC AND PRACTICE ROOM

1. **Keep implements and supplies accessible and orderly.**

    It is important that a system be established and maintained for checking implements and supplies in and out of the supply room. A good system will help keep losses and waste at an absolute minimum. Either a check or requisition system could be created but, whatever the system, provision must be made for keeping careful check and control over materials and supplies.

    Good or poor work habits are formed in the school. If students are trained to respect and control the use of materials and supplies, this training will be carried over into the salon. Cutting down on waste is an important consideration in the beauty salon and beauty school.

2. **Keep equipment and implements in good condition.**

    Any equipment which is not in good working order is not contributing to the educational program. All implements and equipment must be kept in proper working condition at all times. Required repairs should be done without delay in order that maximum teaching and learning benefits be derived.

    Inspection and adjustment of equipment should be a routine matter. Students must be imbued with the importance of maintaining salon equipment at maximum efficiency.

3. **Develop a definite program for maintaining a clean, orderly clinic and work room.**

    Assign specific duties to students in order to maintain a good, clean, orderly clinic. This procedure will make the entire project simple, with no burden on any one student. Keep checking in order to be certain that students are performing properly and forming proper habits for good salon maintenance.

4. **Create a clinic personnel organization.**

    A student organization can be set up which not only will give students an opportunity to assume responsibility but also relieve instructors of a great deal of routine work. A typical student personnel organization of salon manager, desk clerk, safety inspector, sanitation inspector and stock room clerk may be used successfully by instructors. Specific duties are assigned for each job and students are selected for, and rotated in, each position.

5. **Prevent waste of materials and supplies.**

    As an instructor, you can perform a real service both to your students and school if you try to prevent the waste of materials and supplies. Forming proper habits in this area will be of great value to your students in the general practice of cosmetology.

6. **Provide storage space for unfinished practice work.**

    You must supervise the storage of unfinished practice work of your students. The space or area provided for mannequins, wigs, etc. should be accessible to your students, yet safe from tampering, damage and theft.

7. **Create and enforce proper rules and regulations.**

    Do not create unnecessary and burdensome rules but only those which will contribute to the teaching-learning situation.

    Rules should be stated positively, and in simple, understandable language. Students should be advised of the reason for each rule and should be able to see its reasonableness and purpose. They must be made to understand how it contributes to the benefit of all students.

    Whatever rules are made, insist that they be properly obeyed by all students, at all times. Play no favorites and live up to the rules yourself. Keep your list of rules up-to-date and as soon as one has outlived its usefulness, remove it from the list. If this is not done, students become confused as to those which must be obeyed and those to be disregarded.

    For example, if rules require that protective gloves or goggles be used when performing certain tasks, and students are permitted to work without them, then laxity is encouraged.

    Take time during an orientation or lecture period to read and explain all rules and why they are necessary. Students often believe that such rules are unimportant, unnecessarily restrictive, or a whim on the part of the teacher, unless they receive careful explanation of the reasons. Avoid making rules just for the sake of making them; always have a good reason for each one.

8. **Make certain that light is adequate.**

    Students must be able to see in order to function properly. Check to make certain that each student has sufficient light for the work being performed. If you feel that the light is inadequate, check with a light meter. Students will feel more confident, and try harder, if you make it clear that you are interested in their health and welfare.

    If you find that the lighting is insufficient, contact the school management and strongly urge improvement.

9. **Make certain that heat and ventilation are proper for the comfort of students.**

    Ventilation and heat are not always easily controlled but you should exert every effort to insure proper working conditions. Some control may be exercised over temperature by opening and closing windows. At times, temperature changes so gradually that teachers are not aware of it. When this happens, students may become either sleepy or cold. Check the thermometer occasionally and observe student actions.

10. **Requisition only necessary equipment and supplies.**

    Be careful to request only those items required for good teaching. It is always wise to maintain a perpetual inventory of supplies and materials. Do not wait until you are out of an item before re-ordering. Necessary supplies, etc., must never reach the point of complete depletion. The efficiency of the instructor may be judged by the control of adequate materials and supplies at all times.

11. **Keep students busy during entire period.**

    Eliminate any idle time on the part of students. Such time is nonproductive in the teaching-learning cycle. Provide a sufficient program and enough work so that no student, however fast, can complete the entire project and then have nothing to do. Clinic and practice time are very valuable. Usually there is not enough of this time for each student, so do not waste any of it.

12. **Clinic and practice room should be laid out for maximum efficiency.**

    Arrange the physical equipment for the greatest benefit to your students. In arranging equipment, keep in mind the following; safety, adequacy of light and heat, grouping of equipment for efficient handling, production flow and availability to students.

MAINTAINING PROPER RECORDS

1. **Know the characteristics of good records.**

    All forms employed in the school should be simple to maintain and understand. All records must be readily available at all times. Records must be complete and supply all necessary information. Entries should be carefully made and must be legible to anyone reading them. Sufficient space should be provided so that entries can be made easily and clearly.

    All records must have a definite purpose. Recording unneccesary data and information does not add to the educational program and may interfere with the performance of more important duties.

2. **Refer to personal records of students.**

    It is most helpful to the sincere, professional teacher to have knowledge of each student's background of experience and interests. The personal records maintained by the school should supply this information concerning each student.

3. **Records should be meaningful.**

    Records kept by the instructor should be those which contribute to the efficiency of activities in the school. Records frequently required in the clinic include those concerning student kits, lockers, textbooks, workbooks, accidents, attendance, tardiness, passes, student's clinic and practice room activities and reference material.

4. **Maintain permanent records of equipment and supplies.**

   Individual record cards should be maintained for each piece of large equipment. These record cards should be complete in every detail for the particular piece of equipment.

   Perpetual inventory records of supplies provide a check on the amount used and help to eliminate the possibility of running out of material by providing for automatic re-ordering reminders.

5. **Student's progress record.**

   In order to measure teaching effectiveness, it is necessary to have a record of the accomplishments of each student. Services performed by students in the clinic and in the practice room should be carefully recorded. Comment can be made on a daily basis of the quality of the student work performed for future reference.

6. **Minimize record keeping during clinic activity periods.**

   Teachers should be supervising, advising and teaching, not record keeping, while students are engaged in clinic activities. Record systems should be so prepared and designed that they require an absolute minimum amount of time taken from teaching.

7. **Reports and records should be submitted on time.**

   The school administration requires certain records and reports from teachers in order to prepare necessary school data. These school compilations usually must be prepared to meet certain deadlines. It is, therefore, essential that teachers keep their records up-to-date and submit them and reports without unnecessary delays. Do your part, so that the entire job can be completed within the required designated period.

   It is advisable to keep duplicates of important records and reports as proof of their having been prepared and submitted.

Personal Notations . . .

3

PLANNING AND PRESENTING THE LESSON

The success of any instructor depends, to a great extent, upon his (her) ability to plan and present lessons. Most cosmetology instructors were previously salon operators. As professional cosmetologists, they were concerned primarily with performing each salon technique correctly. As instructors, their primary duty is to teach others the knowledge and skills which they possess.

The importance of planning each lesson cannot be over-emphasized. It is unrealistic to expect that any instructor can go into class unprepared and still be able to teach adequately. Complete preparation is absolutely necessary. Teachers should know exactly what they will teach and how they will teach the subject. The lesson plan should be carefully organized and prepared in order that it may be used as a guide whenever a lesson is presented.

LESSON PLANNING

1. **Subject matter selected should conform with course objectives.**

    The subject matter to be selected must contribute to the knowledge and skills that students are expected to acquire. All instruction must conform with the objectives of the course.

2. **The specific objectives of each lesson must be determined.**

    Each lesson has a definite objective. This aim must be clear-cut and specifically defined.

3. **Subject matter must be arranged in order of learning difficulty.**

   Cosmetology should be taught in such a manner that students can learn step-by-step, from the simple fundamentals to the more difficult ones. Students' confidence in their ability to learn is developed by presenting the easiest teaching points at the beginning of the lesson. More difficult phases of the lesson should be gradually introduced as the lesson progresses, in order to prevent student-frustration.

4. **Sufficient material must be available for lesson.**

   If you happen to have a very bright class, the students may learn the planned subject-matter very quickly. If you plan and prepare for only a minimum lesson, you may find yourself in the embarrassing position of having nothing further to present. The competent instructor prepares more material for presentation than he expects to use, and thus is prepared for any eventuality.

5. **Plan the teaching methods to be employed.**

   The teaching method to be employed depends upon the type of lesson to be taught. Some methods are more effective than others in presenting different types of subject matter. After the subject matter has been selected and organized, it is necessary that you select the method of presentation. A combination of methods is usually more effective than a single one.

   It is much more desirable to vary the method of presentation. Using a variety of devices helps to involve all of the student's learning senses.

   Demonstrations and visual aids utilize the sense of sight. Discussions, questions, answers and explanations involve the sense of hearing. The performance of manipulative techniques, the use of samples and other objects utilize the sense of touch and feel. The senses of taste and smell are not very important in the practice of cosmetology; however, these senses may be profitably employed in other areas.

6. **Select teaching aids for use in program.**

   The qualified teacher is very careful to employ many visual aids to increase the effectiveness of the lesson. It is the teacher's responsibility to develop as many such aids as possible, and to recommend to the school's administration which aids should be purchased and which can be prepared in the school.

   Some of the visual aids most commonly used in schools of beauty culture are:

Implements	Chalk Boards	Workbooks
Equipment	Flip Charts	Textbooks
Cosmetic Supplies	Procedure Boards	Motion Pictures
Wall Charts	Pictures	Film Strips
Diagrams	Posters	Slides
Models	Notebooks	Projectors
Mock-ups	Mannequins	Transparencies

7. **Develop means to obtain student participation.**

   In order for teaching and learning to be effective, activity on the part of the students is required. You, as an instructor, must develop as much student activity and participation as possible.

   Most of the student's time in the practice room and clinic is devoted to manual activity. Students learn best when they use their hands and eyes, as well as their minds, in any learning situation.

   Some of the methods commonly used to encourage student participation are:
   a) Asking questions.
   b) Encouraging students to ask questions.
   c) Use of the chalk board.
   d) Studentes' participation in demonstrations.
   e) Students' helping in making and using visual aids.
   f) Class discussions.

8. **Plan method of motivating students.**

   As a professional instructor you must not only carefully prepare each lesson in advance, but must also prepare your students to receive it. The teacher plans to motivate the students' desire to learn the material. Usually the reason for failure of students to learn is the fact that they are not sufficiently interested, and not that they lack ability.

   It is essential that you arouse the interest of your students in the subject matter to be presented. They must be informed of the importance of the lesson, how the material applies to the over-all objective of the course and the importance of the material in contributing to their success as cosmetologists.

   You must not be so interested in trying to drive home the technical information that you forget the interest factor. Relate some of your own experiences where the information was important. Ask students for their own beauty salon experiences which might apply. The interest factor is a most important essential to learning.

9. **Recommend references for further study.**

   You must always be prepared to recommend sources for further study, if students express or indicate interest to further study a particular subject. A list of references should be included in your lesson plan, and made available to all students.

10. **Plan first session for student orientation.**

    The first day in school is of vital importance to every new student. Many first impressions create attitudes which affect the future conduct of students. The first day should be designed to put students at ease, make them feel comfortable in their new surroundings and implant a desire for learning.

Orientation of new students should be so planned as to arouse interest and develop an understanding of the school and its functions. The over-all objective, to train students to become professional cosmetologists, should be explained and students indoctrinated with the thought that all student activities are designed to meet that one objective.

Cosmetology student orientation should include:
a) A broad discussion of the over-all aims and objectives of the entire program.
b) A brief description of the class room program, practice room and clinic activities; and the importance of each of these in the development of the overall program.
c) Distribution of kits and explaining their contents.
d) An explanation of the school rules and regulations.
e) The class schedule to be followed.
f) How students are graded and evaluated.
g) Assignment of students to teachers and practice room stations.

11. **Provide for the explanation and definition of new cosmetology words and phrases.**

Students cannot be expected to absorb and learn new material if they are not familiar with the words and phrases used. You must never assume that your students understand the new technical words.

It is advisable that each lesson include a list of the new technical words used, with an explanation and definition of each. In presenting a lesson to your class, test constantly to be certain that you are being understood.

12. **Summarize your lesson.**

Every lesson should include a summary of the important points covered. Select the important points as part of your lesson plan and conduct a brief review in order to help your students to organize the material in their own minds and in their notes. A workbook is an excellent device to use for review.

13. **Good education includes ample testing.**

Before presenting new material, it is important that you are certain that your students have understood and learned the subject matter just taught. This may be done in various ways, such as giving oral quizzes, asking questions, giving written examinations, or checking and observing manual performance and dexterity in the practice room or clinic.

14. **Plan new assignments for students.**

New study assignments must be planned in advance as part of your lesson plan. Make sure that your assignments are clear and specific and that your students understand clearly what is expected of them.

PREPARING THE LESSON PLAN

1. **Create a descriptive title for the lesson.**

    Each lesson plan should have a title which is descriptive of the subject matter to be taught. For example, the title of a classroom lesson could be:

    "The Action of the Solution in Permanent Waving," or "Wrapping Cold Wave Curls."

2. **Time to be devoted to the lesson should be stated.**

    Each lesson should include information as to the length of time to be devoted to it. Time is planned carefully to cover the material to be presented and also to fit into the over-all allocation of time for the entire course.

    This information is essential to avoid interference with other subjects and to advise all instructors teaching the particular subject of the time to be spent on it.

3. **Lesson plans must be flexible.**

    No lesson plan should be so prepared that it's inflexible. Cosmetology is a rapidly changing vocation and schools must keep alert as to new developments and ideas. Lesson plans should be under constant study for revision and improvement. Whenever improvements and changes are made in methods or techniques, the lesson plans should be revised to incorporate such changes.

4. **Be thoroughly prepared before class.**

    The well prepared lesson plan contains a list of all materials, visual aids and other instructional data to be used in the presentation. You must be certain that all such materials have been collected, and are in good condition, before the class meets. Refer to your lesson plan and check to be certain that all necessary preparations have been made.

5. **Refer to lesson plan frequently during presentation.**

    The lesson plan should be used as a guide in presenting a lesson. Refer to it as often as necessary during the presentation and development of the lesson to make certain that nothing is overlooked.

6. **Form of lesson plan.**

    There is a stock form available which lists all items required for a lesson plan. It is designed to include everything which is needed for a particular job. Sample may be obtained from:

    Milady Publishing Corp.
    3839 White Plains Road
    Bronx, New York, 10467

LESSON PLAN OUTLINE

The following list is presented as a guide in the preparation of a good lesson plan. It should be followed to be certain that the lesson plan is prepared as an effective and comprehensive teaching aid.

Outline

1. Create a descriptive title.
2. State objectives of lesson.
3. Allocate and state time to be devoted.
4. List teaching aids to be used.
5. Indicate the method of presentation.
6. Plan your motivation—arouse student interest.
7. Method for stimulating student participation.
8. List new words and phrases with definitions.
9. Statement of subject matter to be covered.
10. Summary and review.
11. Provide for testing—list of questions.
12. For practical work, provide for practice session.
13. Student assignments.
14. Additional sources of reference.

PRESENTATION OF LESSON

1. **Use lesson plan as guide.**

    The lesson plan is the instructor's road map of ground to be covered. It directs the presentation of the subject matter and the order in which each item is to be taken up. The wise instructor refers to his lesson plan without hesitation, in order to be certain that his presentation is accurate and complete.

2. **Arouse and maintain student interest.**

    A cosmetology instructor is not employed to entertain his students. However, the teacher who is enthusiastic, peppy and animated transfers this enthusiasm to the class. You will have little difficulty in arousing your students if you employ a bit of humor occasionally; in other words, use a little showmanship in order to arouse and maintain the interest of your students.

3. **Stand while presenting lesson.**

    An instructor must be able to see all students and observe their reactions to the presentation of the subject matter. He cannot properly and clearly see all students while sitting at a desk. Every instructor can do a much better job while standing, since the students can see him and he has a clear view of the entire class.

4. **Talk directly to your class.**

    The competent instructor faces the class at all times. You will be better understood if you talk directly to your students and not to a chalk board or off into space. Be sure that you speak clearly in order that all students can hear and understand you.

5. **Before leaving any point, be certain that the entire class understands it.**

    Make certain that your class understands each point covered. This can be done by asking questions. Do not depend upon your "ability to read faces." A few well chosen questions will help to determine how well the class has absorbed your presentation.

6. **Do not hold up group progress for the few who do not understand.**

    If you spend too much time explaining and re-explaining the subject matter to a few slow-learning students, the balance of the class will lose interest and become restless. It is wiser to continue with the class and make some special provision to supply additional teaching to the slower students. This might be accomplished by planning some constructive, challenging work for your brighter students, while giving extra attention to the slow ones.

7. **Taking notes must be constructive.**

    Require your students to take notes only when they will prove useful. Notes should involve recording the essential points of a lesson as an aid to organizing information and providing review material for study prior to tests, or for future reference.

    It is neither constructive nor educationally sound to dictate long notes or to have students copy material from the chalk board. Cosmetology instructors should not form the habit of creating work just to keep students busy. Every task must serve an important purpose in the over-all objective of the course.

8. **The use of the "workbook."**

    Cosmetology instructors and students will find the use of workbooks to be very valuable for drill work and review study. The workbook presents an organized arrangement of subject matter in which students can exercise their understanding of classroom material. The workbook gives instructors a very comprehensive area for out-of-class assignments.

Personal Notations . . .

30

CONDUCTING DEMONSTRATIONS

One of the most effective methods employed in teaching cosmetology is the demonstration. It is possible to teach the manipulative techniques of cosmetology by several different methods. However, the most effective of these is by actually showing students how the work is done. Students not only learn faster but also retain the technique longer when they learn by seeing. It is, therefore, important that the cosmetology teacher master the art of presenting a good demonstration.

PREPARING FOR THE DEMONSTRATION

1. **Planned demonstrations should not be too lengthy.**

    Demonstrations should not be conducted over too long a period of time. They should not include too many operations, since students may become tired or confused and may not remember all the techniques shown and explained.

    Demonstrations must be carefully planned in advance. The instructor must be thoroughly familiar with each technique. If you are at all uncertain concerning any part of the demonstration, then practice before class, in order to perform flawlessly.

    If any demonstration appears too long, then it is advisable to break it up into a series of short demonstrations. In that event, make certain that there is a clearly defined continuity of the operations. If there is any break in the continuity, the entire series becomes worthless and a waste of time. Short demonstrations are usually the best for teaching and learning.

2. **Prepare all materials, equipment and supplies in advance.**

   Before starting a demonstration be certain that you have accumulated all necessary materials and supplies. The complete effectiveness of a demonstration is destroyed if the instructor is suddenly required to stop and leave the classroom to obtain some necessary instrument or supplies. All equipment, instruments, supplies and material must be readily available and properly arranged before the demonstration starts.

3. **Develop interest by explaining objectives of the demonstration.**

   The qualified cosmetology instructor first explains the importance of the demonstration. All students should be fully informed as to how the technique they are to witness fits into salon practice, and the importance of acquiring the ability to do it properly. The specific objectives of the demonstration should be explained and students' interest aroused so that they are eager to learn.

4. **Brief students in advance on important points.**

   Students should be given a brief preview of the highlights of the demonstration. This is done in order that they have an idea of what to expect and the important points they are to look for.

PERFORMANCE OF THE DEMONSTRATION

1. **Explain new words, terms and techniques.**

   Be certain that your students understand any new words or terms that you are using as part of the demonstration. Explain any new techniques you are introducing. Make your explanation clear and detailed in order that all students understand.

2. **Supplement demonstration with visual aids.**

   Whenever possible, supplement your demonstration with visual teaching aids. The use of such visual aids will make your demonstration more clearly understood and will add interest to it. Some of the usual visual aids used for this purpose are: charts, flip charts, diagrams, pictures, cutaways and samples.

3. **Each student must be able to see and hear clearly.**

   Arrange your class and your demonstration so that each student has a clear, unobstructed view. If students cannot see or hear, the entire demonstration is a waste of time. If necessary, divide a large class into small groups and repeat the demonstration in order to obtain maximum effectiveness.

4. **Face students and talk directly to them.**

    Demonstrations should be so set up that the instructor can see each student and be able to talk directly to the entire group. Never arrange your class in such a way that some students will be unable to see, hear or participate.

5. **Associate demonstration with earlier and future lessons.**

    It is advisable that the instructor associate the demonstration with work previously learned and with techniques to be taught in the future. Student interest will be aroused more easily if they understand the relationship of the demonstration to skills they have already acquired or to techniques which they will be expected to learn for beauty salon work.

6. **Pace demonstration for maximum learning efficiency.**

    Make sure that each technique is performed slowly enough so that each movement is clearly seen and understood by all students. Each operation should be thoroughly explained as it is being performed.

7. **Each technique must be performed skillfully and in correct sequence.**

    In order to be effective the techniques and procedures of the demonstration should be skillfully performed. If you, the instructor, are to set professional standards for your students, you must perform before them with proper professional skill. The opportunity is afforded to the instructor to actually demonstrate the proper standards of work performance. It also gives the opportunity to build up the confidence of students in their own ability to perform by having them repeat the technique after the demonstration is completed under his supervision.

8. **The progress of the entire class should not be held up by a few slow students.**

    Demonstrations are intended to accomplish the greatest good for the greatest number of students. The progress of many should not be retarded by a few slow students. The demonstration should be completed for the entire group and then slower students should be brought back for further explanations and training.

9. **Test understanding, during demonstration, by asking questions.**

    At frequent intervals during the demonstration, the instructor should ask questions, to test understanding. Because some students are shy or do not wish to appear foolish, they will rarely volunteer a question. To combat this, the instructor should ask questions.

    A question should always require definite answers; not "yes" or "no."

10. **Students should be encouraged to ask questions at any time.**

    The instructor must develop an understanding of those areas most difficult to learn. In order to discover these areas, students should be encouraged to ask questions at any time during the demonstration.

    Students must be made to realize that no question is foolish, if it is asked sincerely, with a desire for understanding. All questions should be accepted seriously and answered thoroughly.

11. **Sanitation and safety precautions must be stressed throughout demonstration.**

    The instructor must make it a special point to stress the safe and correct way for performing every operation. Careless cosmetologists are liabilities to themselves and to their employers, no matter how skillful they may be.

    Personal injuries and damage to equipment are costly, and every effort must be taken to avoid them. Accidents are usually caused; they do not "just happen." Students must be carefully taught to prevent accidents.

    The instructor must practice sanitation in order that students observe the sanitary measures which must be followed.

12. **Enlist students to assist with demonstration, if possible.**

    Upon completion of the demonstration, it often is advisable to select a student to repeat the entire performance. This technique helps to test understanding of the demonstration and arouses the interest of the entire class. Students usually watch the performance of their fellow-student with great interest. Many times they become more interested and absorbed in the student's performance than they were in the teacher's.

COMPLETION OF DEMONSTRATION

1. **Emphasize important points.**

    A brief review or summary of the important points of the demonstration will serve to emphasize these areas.

2. **Question and answer period.**

    After the completion of the demonstration, it would be a good policy to conduct a quiz in order to determine whether or not the essential areas have been clearly understood.

3. **Plan for student practice immediately following demonstration.**

    While the process demonstrated is clearly outlined in students' minds, they should be assigned to practice the techniques taught.

This practice helps to solidify the learning process and to maintain high student interest.

Work assignments should be given before the start of the demonstration in order that they start without any delay.

4. **Each student's work should be examined and checked.**

A good cosmetology instructor follows a demonstration with personalized instruction. Circulate among the students; observe their work and techniques; ask questions; check their understanding, and prevent formation of poor work habits by immediate correction. This procedure is of great assistance to the instructor in testing the effectiveness of the demonstration and in locating areas of teaching or learning weakness.

5. **Study assignments for students.**

New study assignments is the final part of your lesson plan, which must be prepared in advance.

Good lesson planning calls for assignments that are clear, meaningful, and, therefore, interesting to students. They should include textbook and workbook pages.

Personal Notations . . .

5

THE USE OF ORAL QUESTIONING TO MAKE TEACHING MORE EFFECTIVE

USES OF ORAL QUESTIONING

The question and answer method is effective in teaching cosmetology. The instructor's ability to use this method properly is one of the elements of good teaching. This teaching technique may be used effectively for many purposes, such as:

1. To motivate the student.
2. To find out the students' interests, abilities and knowledge.
3. To encourage student participation.
4. To review and summarize the important points in a lesson.
5. To arouse interest and direct attention of students to a particular area.
6. To clarify a point.
7. To stimulate discussion and confine it to a certain subject.
8. To spot check effectiveness of instruction.
9. To stress a point.
10. To retain attention.
11. To assist students in planning their work and analyzing their problems.
12. To test students' knowledge and understanding, and thus evaluate the effectiveness of the teaching.

1. **All students should be required to speak so they can be heard.**

   Insist that students speak loudly enough to be heard by the entire class. If anyone in the class cannot hear, the student should be asked to speak louder. Interest soon lags if students cannot hear clearly.

2. **Use correct grammar.**

   For effective instruction, every teacher should use correct grammar and try to improve his use of English in order that he be better understood. The instructor should also insist that students use proper English.

3. **Use simple language.**

   In order to make your questioning effective, use common words that can be understood by all students. Do not talk over the heads of your class or fail to explain words which they do not readily understand.

4. **Questions should be confined to subject.**

   The tendency to wander from the prime subject is one of the difficulties of the discussion method. Students may ask questions which direct the discussion into foreign channels. The effective instructor carefully guides the discussion in order to keep questions confined to the subject matter.

5. **Questions should be part of a definite plan.**

   The instructor should direct questions toward a specific objective and according to a definite plan. A list of questions should be part of the lesson plan, in order to be certain that they be asked at the proper time and in proper relation to each other.

6. **Questions should require thought.**

   Although some questions may simply ask a student to repeat from memory, it is more effective to provide questions that require the application of the material being taught. For this reason, problem questions are particularly good.

   Questions that can be answered "yes" or "no" are of little value. All questions should be pertinent and should stimulate thought on the part of the students before they can answer. Use "how," "why," and "what" when asking questions. To be successful as an instructor you must master the art of creating questions such as:

   a) Why do we do it?
   b) What is its purpose?
   c) Where should it be done?
   d) When should it be done?
   e) Who should do it?
   f) How should it be done?
   g) Which is the better technique?

7. **Questions should be brief and easily understood.**

   It is poor teaching to ask questions which are tricky or which may be interpreted in several ways. All questions should be so stated that students clearly understand them and know exactly what is expected. If it is apparent that students do not understand a question, it should be rephrased immediately in words which will be understood.

8. **Procedure for questioning.**

   First ask the question of the entire class. Pause to give everyone a chance to consider the question. Then call upon a student to answer. Select the students at random; otherwise, some students will not pay attention until they think it is their turn.

   Questions should be answered by students only if their names have been called. No answers in unison should be permitted.

9. **Do not repeat questions for inattentive students.**

   A question should immediately be repeated if it is not clear to students. However, never repeat the question for a student who has been inattentive.

10. **Ask only questions which can be answered.**

    Questions should be asked which stimulate thinking and discussion; however, they must not be too difficult for students to answer. If no one can answer the question, the instructor should immediately restate it, in more easily understood terms or ask an easier question.

11. **Only individual responses should be permitted.**

    At the very beginning of the course, the instructor should explain the accepted procedure for students to follow in answering questions. It must be made very clear that only individual responses will be accepted and only when directed by the instructor.

12. **Students should never be called upon in rotation.**

    Questioning students in rotation, according to alphabetical names or seating, reduces the participation and attention of the entire class. Students become aware of when their turn will come and, as a result, may become inactive and inattentive until they are about to be called.

13. **Students should be called upon with reasonable frequency.**

    In order to permit the instructor to test the understanding of all students, they should be called upon with reasonable frequency. It also helps the instructor to become better acquainted with the students as individuals.

14. **If possible, questions should fit each individual student.**

    The efficient instructor will make every effort to understand the members of the class. This will permit the teacher to ask less difficult questions of slower students and more difficult questions of brighter students, thus contributing to the effectiveness of the question and answer method of teaching.

15. **Students should answer from their seats.**

    Students should not be required to stand when answering questions, since this may prove embarrassing to some students and affect their ability to answer. It is the aim of the question and discussion method to secure reactions from all students and this can be better accomplished when they are permitted to speak from their seats.

16. **All students should be encouraged to participate.**

    The good instructor encourages students to ask reasonable questions pertaining to the subject matter at any time. The instructor should give serious consideration to, and answer all questions. However, if the instructor does not know the answer he should honestly admit that fact and should try to find the answer.

    When asking questions, allow a reasonable time for students to think before they answer.

    Do not permit a few students to monopolize the discussion.

    Call on students whose minds are wandering to bring them back to the subject matter and to stimulate their thinking.

    Never embarrass students with speech impediments or other physical ailments.

17. **Be careful not to give clues to answers by facial expressions.**

    In order to make the most efficient use of the questioning method, the instructor must be careful not to indicate answers by gestures, leading words, facial expressions, etc. Student-thinking may be considerably reduced by a teacher who gives clues to answers.

18. **Refrain from injecting personal references.**

    Comments referring to personal qualities of students or other instructors are not part of the lesson plan and should be avoided. All discussions should avoid any personal or uncomplimentary statements or remarks.

19. **Arrive at a definite conclusion to a discussion.**

    Every discussion program must be carefully planned and guided by the instructor. It is important to crystallize the important points of the discussion and arrive at definite conclusions. Discussions should never be ended unless conclusions have been developed. The instructor should carefully summarize the high points of the lesson and help students to formulate conclusions and understanding.

20. **Oral Questions Check List** YES NO

   a) Did the questions motivate the students? .... ☐ ☐

   b) Did the questions find out what students already knew? .... ☐ ☐

   c) Did the questions encourage active participation of students? .... ☐ ☐

   d) Did questions spot check quality of instruction? ☐ ☐

   e) Did questions help to clarify points students had not previously understood? .... ☐ ☐

   f) Did questions serve to stress important points? ☐ ☐

   g) Did questions help hold the attention of the students? .... ☐ ☐

   h) Did questions help to review material taught? ☐ ☐

   i) Were questions brief and easily understood? .... ☐ ☐

   j) Did questions require thought? .... ☐ ☐

   k) Was each question limited to one primary idea? ☐ ☐

   l) Did each question have a specific purpose which was related to the subject under discussion? .... ☐ ☐

   m) Did the instructor ask the questions and then name students to answer? .... ☐ ☐

Personal Notations . . .

THE USE OF AUDIO-VISUAL AIDS

Teaching and learning should take place every minute while the student is in school.

The formal teaching presentations of course, are the principal factors in student progress in the curriculum areas. However, such lessons are far from the only factors by which students learn.

The example set by the instructor's manner, attitude, appearance, readiness, actions, voice, etc., constitute an endless lesson that has a tremendous impact on student learning.

The actions of each student and the responses to such actions by the teacher and fellow students all create learning situations.

Each of the innumerable classroom situations that occur in a learning atmosphere, whether it will be a negative or a positive one, depends on the skill of the teacher in utilizing spontaneous opportunities for learning.

One of the most effective methods employed by modern instructors in their efforts is the use of audio-visual aids.

TEACHING AND LEARNING ADVANTAGES TO BE DERIVED FROM SLIDES, FILMS, FILM-STRIPS AND TRANSPARENCIES

Earlier discussions stressed the importance of the use of the several senses to make learning more effective. Audio-visual aids help to accomplish this objective. Furthermore, some things are difficult to describe just by using words, but can be understood clearly when seen.

Most students learn easily and quickly through the sense of sight. Presenting students with a "visual image" of any technique eliminates the necessity for building their own "mental image" from the words used by the instructor. The picture itself is presented more quickly, and is understood more clearly, than are written or spoken words.

"A picture is worth a thousand words." A picture of the real thing is next best to the actual thing. Under some conditions a picture may be a better learning device than the real thing. Therefore, the use of films, film-strips, slides and transparencies are often more effective teaching aids than the object itself.

The following suggestions are offered as guides for the use of audio-visual aids.

PREPARATION FOR USE

1. **Audio-visual aids must not be used as substitutes for the teacher.**

    In using audio-visual aids the instructor must carefully prepare the lesson in advance. These items are most effective only when using them as aids in teaching. They are of little or no value when merely used as substitutes for the teacher's own initiative.

2. **Films, slides, film-strips or transparencies should not be used if a more effective method is available.**

    Audio-visual equipment is not a "cure-all" for all teaching weaknesses. Simply because the aid is available does not automatically mean that it must be used. The instructor must analyze carefully the various methods of presenting the lesson and reject audio-visual equipment if other methods or devices may prove more successful.

3. **Films, slides and transparencies are not to be used to entertain students.**

    Instructors must exert every effort to orient students to the use and purpose of educational films, slides and transparencies. Students should be made to understand clearly that they are being used for the sole purpose of helping them to learn, and under no circumstances are they to be considered as an entertainment feature. It is the teacher's responsibility to use the aids as truly instructional devices.

4. **Carefully plan timing for use of aid.**

    The teacher should schedule the use of the aid at a point where it can make a specific and pertinent contribution to the teaching-learning situation.

    A film, film-strip, transparencies or series of slides may be very helpful when presented at the beginning of a program for teaching a particular technique. If the visual aid were presented after the students had been taught the technique, had worked with it and had become thoroughly familiar with its performance, its value to a large degree, would be wasted.

5. **The teacher must preview audio-visual aids before presentation to class.**

    The instructor must preview the films, film-strips, transparencies or slide series; pre-listen to recordings; consult guidebooks and in other ways assure himself of their content.

    Titles are often misleading and frequently the content is unsatisfactory. Only those audio-visual aids which contribute to the course objectives should be selected for use.

6. **Carefully prepare a lesson plan for presentation.**

    A detailed lesson plan should be prepared as a guide for the presentation of the audio-visual aid. This lesson plan should include:
    a) Title of lesson
    b) Objectives
    c) Time required
    d) Other items to supplement audio-visual aids
    e) Instructional aids
    f) Means for developing student interest
    g) Devices for securing student participation
    h) Explanations of new terms
    i) Statement of important points to look for
    j) Remarks to supplement visual presentation
    k) Important points for summary
    l) Methods for testing student-understanding
    m) Assignments
    n) References for additional study and reading

7. **Prepare study guide for students.**

    A study guide for students can be of great value when presenting films as teaching aids. The guide should list the title of the film, the objectives of the lesson, and an explanation of new terms and important points to look for. It should also contain a list of questions, to be answered by students, based upon the film. Questions should also be prepared for classroom discussion.

    It is wise to include reference material for outside study and for discussion at future classes.

8. **Students should be seated so that all can see and hear clearly.**

    The classroom should be arranged in such a manner that all students can see the screen, and hear the entire presentation, without any interference.

9. **Focus projector before class.**

    It is the instructor's responsibility to properly set up the projector before the class meets. The projector should be threaded, focused and tested in advance. The instructor must be capable of properly using the projector without unnecessary delay.

    The effectiveness of the entire program could be destroyed by improper use of the equipment.

10. **Lighting conditions must be tested.**

    The lighting arrangements in the room must be properly adjusted to permit the best results.

    When using a film strip or slides, there should be sufficient light in the room to permit the teacher to see all students and for the students to see the instructor.

    When using a film, the room should be darkened for best results.

11. **Adequate ventilation must be provided.**

    The use of curtains, shades, closed doors and other devices employed to darken the room may all cut down on ventilation. It is important, therefore, that the instructor make every effort to be certain that proper ventilation is provided in some fashion.

12. **All preparations must be made before class.**

    A good instructor will prepare all teaching material before the class meets. All hand-outs, study guides, etc., must be on hand before the start of the class.

    The projector must be ready for use, and seating, lighting and other necessary arrangements made in advance.

PRESENTATION OF FILMS

1. **Prepare students.**

    Before running any cosmetology film, the students must be properly prepared to receive it.

    The teacher should first explain, to the class, the objective in presenting the film. A brief explanation should be given of the contents of the film. Each student should receive a study guide. Interest must be aroused in the educational and learning benefits to be derived. Students are advised to look for certain important points, and new words and phrases are explained. Students should be informed in advance that they will be required to answer questions on the contents of the film.

2. **Run through entire film.**

It is good teaching practice to first run through the entire film without stopping.

This practice permits students to obtain a complete view of the entire operation. It gives them an understanding of the relationships between the various operations and processes demonstrated.

3. **Re-run parts or entire film for clarification.**

In order to clarify or expand on difficult phases of the work demonstrated, the instructor could re-run part or all of the film.

4. **Instructor's comments should supplement film.**

In order to clarify and help students to understand points not covered by captions, the instructor should make pertinent remarks at various points in the demonstration. However, when showing a sound picture, absolutely no remarks should be made by the instructor, lest he detract from the learning pattern created by the film.

5. **Instructor should stand or sit in back of room.**

For proper teaching with films, the instructor should stand or sit at the rear of the room. He is thus able to observe the entire class more clearly and be quickly available if anything goes wrong. The instructor is also in a better position to maintain classroom discipline.

6. **Avoid delays in changing reels.**

If unnecessary or prolonged delays occur due to the changing of reels or mechanical difficulties, a great deal of student-interest may be lost. Therefore, every precaution should be taken to prevent these delays. However, should they occur, interest could be maintained by a short discussion on what has already been shown, while the condition is being remedied.

PRESENTATION OF FILM-STRIPS

1. **Prepare students.**

Students must be properly prepared to receive the film-strip and their interest aroused. They must understand in advance the objective to be obtained from the film-strip. They must be mentally, emotionally and physically ready to watch the presentation and accept it with relation to course objectives.

2. **Teacher must stand in front of class.**

It is essential that the instructor stand in front of the class when presenting film-strips. The teacher must face the entire class if he (she) wishes to present a lesson effectively, and must talk directly to the class in order to obtain and keep its interest and attention.

When using film-strips, the instructor should make it a point to direct student attention to certain important areas. He (she) may also wish to supplement the film-strip with short demonstrations or by the use of other teaching devices. All of these require that the instructor remain in front of the class during the entire lesson.

3. **Make use of captions of frames as teaching instruments.**

    The wise instructor capitalizes on and uses the captions of the individual frames as teaching instruments.

    He reads aloud the caption of each frame, emphasizing certain words or phrases. He injects important remarks into the reading of the captions and makes certain that the students understand each point. The instructor thus is able to obtain the widest possible use of the film strip as a teaching device.

4. **Point out important parts of film-strip.**

    By using a long pointer, the instructor may indicate important parts of each image. The pointer helps focus attention to the exact area which is receiving special attention.

5. **For clarification, make comments of certain frames.**

    In order to increase the effectiveness of the film-strip, the good instructor makes comments and offers explanations in addition to the film captions. Brief remarks about the correct application of the material shown in the film, an explanation of certain unclear frames and other pertinent comments can add greatly to the effectiveness of the presentation.

6. **Question students during presentation.**

    It is highly recommended that instructors frequently employ the use of questions during film-strip presentations. This procedure encourages students to participate in the discussions, stimulates their thinking, holds their attention and presents the instructor with a means of testing for undersanding.

7. **Film-strips with commentary.**

    If the film-strip has its own commentary the instructor should wait until it has run through, before making statements, asking questions or starting discussions of its contents.

PRESENTATION OF SLIDES

1. **Slides are very effective in cosmetology training.**

    The use of a series of slides in a cosmetology training lesson brings a very effective visual-aid to the classroom. It gives every benefit of a film-strip and also permits a longer and detailed instructional breakdown.

2. **Permits additions and deletions from series.**

    A slide series has the distinct advantage of permitting the addition or deletion of certain slides whenever desired. It also permits rearrangement of the slides to improve instruction.

3. **Permits instructor to make own slides.**

    The instructor should find it relatively simple to make his or her own slides of a particular cosmetology technique which it is especially desirable to present in this manner.

4. **Preparation and presentation of slides similar to those for film-strips.**

    All suggestions offered for the preparation and presentation of film-strips must be applied to the presentation of a slide series.

5. **Slides permit the halting at single slide for detailed discussion.**

    When presenting a slide series, it is sometimes desirable to stop at a particular slide for lengthy discussion. The instructor can point out important areas for detailed study. In fact, a single slide may form the basis for a complete lesson.

6. **Slides offer an ideal method for presenting a new technique and also, for review.**

    A slide series can be most helpful to the cosmetology teacher in presenting a new technique. It could develop a step-by-step presentation of the procedure to be taught. The slides also could be employed as a method for reviewing an entire manipulative procedure.

7. **Characteristics of a good audio-visual aid.**

    An audio-visual aid is a specifically prepared device which will expedite learning through the senses of both sight and hearing. When selecting or making an audio-visual aid, the following points should be considered:

    a) It should explain an idea, show a relationship or present a sequence or procedure in a most effective manner.
    b) It should be large enough to be seen and heard clearly by everyone in the class.
    c) The lettering should be large and bold, to avoid eyestrain from any point in the room.
    d) The wording should be easy for the students to understand.
    e) The important areas should be accentuated in some way.
    f) It should be constructed of good material, so that it can be used frequently.
    g) It should be portable, to permit its use in more than one location.
    h) It should be used as an aid to teaching, not as a substitute for the teacher.

PRESENTATION OF TRANSPARENCIES

The overhead projector is one of the newer visual-aids that has rapidly taken over the role of the opaque projector which performs in a similar manner. Whereas the opaque projector does project materials, such as photographs, magazine pages and other photographed or printed materials, the overhead projector uses clear transparencies and, therefore, provides more brightness and clarity. Furthermore, the modern overhead projector is lightweight and portable which makes its employment a simple matter.

The main advantages of the overhead projector are:

1. **Student eye contact is maintained.**

    With the overhead projector there is no need to worry about what is going on behind your back . . . you never turn away from your students in utilizing this device. This is because the screen is positioned above and behind the instructor and all her attention is focused on the platform of the projector that holds the transparency and on the student whom she is addressing.

2. **It is most suitable for teaching theory and scientific subjects.**

    Since theoretical and scientific subjects do not require a rapid sequence of illustrations, the instructor can pace himself (herself) and dwell as long as necessary on a particular point of information or diagram.

3. **Hairstyling can also be effectively taught by use of the overhead projector.**

    Hairstyling has to do with space, form and patterns. All of these can be illustrated and discussed at length.

4. **Transparencies can be prepared in multiple colors and with multiple overlays.**

    The nature of each transparency permits the use of color which can be quite effective in the presentation of many topics. Furthermore, special overlays can be made up to permit the isolation of single parts of illustrations or used simultaneously to give a complete picture. This builds interest and increases student attention.

5. **It is simple to operate.**

    A simple on-and-off switch and focusing knob are all that are involved in the operation of the device. Furthermore, pointing to individual items on a transparency is achieved without a mechanical device and most instructors will use a pencil or some similar object that will cast a reflected shadow on the transparency and, hence, on the screen.

6. **Commercially prepared transparencies are available.**

    Complete sets of overhead projector transparencies are available to cover all of the major cosmetology subjects, both theoretical and practical.

Furthermore, extensive research has been carried out and suitable overhead projector transparencies have been prepared for teaching the subjects of hair structure and chemistry. For further information write to:

  Milady Publishing Corp.
  3839 White Plains Road
  Bronx, New York, 10467

7. **Teachers can make their own transparencies.**

    Teachers can supplement commercially prepared series by making their own transparencies. Illustrations can be reproduced on certain office copying machines and immediately put into use.

FOLLOWING THE PRESENTATION

Audio-visual aids should never be used without follow-up activities which capitalize on the occasion.

1. **Test for understanding and learning.**

    Some means of testing for student understanding and learning should follow each use of an audio-visual aid. The instructor may use oral questions or a written objective test as effective methods for evaluation.

    The student study guide or workbook are both excellent devices in testing for student understanding; they are also important review implements.

2. **Develop a class discussion of the presentation.**

    The important points covered in the presentation should be reviewed in a class discussion. This method helps to obtain active participation by all students. It also helps the instructor to understand the students and to maintain student interest.

3. **Present summary of lesson.**

    The good instructor will summarize the lesson by emphasizing important areas and pointing out the definite conclusions which have been developed.

4. **Correct any errors or wrong conclusions.**

    If any of the techniques, facts or processes shown are not in complete agreement with the procedure taught in the school, they should be carefully explained in order to avoid misunderstanding and confusion.

5. **If necessary, supplement the presentation by employing other visual-aids.**

    On occasion it may become necessary to further clarify doubtful or difficult areas. This can be done by using other types of visual-aids, after the presentation. A number of other visual-aids, such as, cutaway models, diagrams, chalk board drawings and other devices which apply to the subject can be used to supplement the presentation whenever possible.

USING THE CHALK BOARD

1. **Proper use of the chalk board.**

    Chalk board work should be simple and brief. It is a waste of time, for both students and teacher, to copy lengthy material on the chalk board. If it is important for the students to have the material, it should be duplicated and distributed.

2. **Chalk board is most effective if kept clean and contains few items.**

    The chalk board has little real teaching or learning value if it is overcrowded, dirty or untidy. The chalk board is most effective as a training aid when it is kept clean and neat, and displays only a few well-chosen items.

3. **Rules for increasing effectiveness of chalk board.**
    a) Don't crowd the chalk board. A few important points make a vivid impression.
    b) Make the material simple. Brief, concise statements are more effective than lengthy ones.
    c) Plan chalk board work in advance.
    d) Gather all necessary supplies in advance—chalk, ruler, eraser, etc.
    e) Check lighting to avoid chalk board glare. If necessary, lower shades and put on lights.
    f) Use color for emphasis. Yellow and green chalk may be more effective than white.
    g) Print all captions and drawings in large scale in order that they be clearly visible to all students.
    h) Erase all unrelated material. Other work on the chalk board distracts attention.
    i) Remove materials from chalk board with eraser or cloth; never use your fingers.
    j) Keep the chalk board clean.
    k) Prepare complicated chalk board layouts before the class meets.
    l) Do not turn your back on class while writing on chalk board.

7

THE USE OF EXAMINATIONS (TESTS) IN THE TEACHING PROGRAM

One of the most valuable of teaching and learning aids is the examination. Most people are of the opinion that the sole function of a test is to allocate grades or marks to students. This belief is quite contrary to the actual facts in the educational spectrum. Tests (examinations) are excellent instructional devices; they are used as teaching tools. A wise cosmetology instructor will employ them to discover the actual knowledge of a subject that students have at a particular time and incorporate that knowledge into planning the teaching program.

Like any other good artisan, the instructor is working to achieve specific, measurable results. To decide whether each lesson, series of lessons, or the complete course is successful, the instructor must use tests, since careful evaluation of their results will compare actual learning achievements with the desired objectives.

TESTS EMPLOYED TO DISCOVER WEAKNESSES

Examinations help to discover and correct weaknesses in student learning and teaching weaknesses on the part of the instructor. The tests indicate which areas of a subject have been mastered, while also pointing out those areas requiring additional training and attention. They also provide the instructor with the knowledge necessary to advise poor students that they are not doing well and in which areas they must exercise extra effort if they wish to progress.

EXAMINATIONS EMPLOYED AS STUDY INCENTIVES

Examinations provide students with required incentives to study. Students realize that they will be questioned over a wide area, and not being informed in advance of the questions to be asked, they must study all of the material. Thus, they review all of the information provided in class and try to organize the material for any eventuality. Tests, therefore, instigate additional study and learning in order to obtain good marks.

TESTING USED TO ESTABLISH STANDARDS

Instructors employ tests in order to compare the quantity and quality of the subject matter absorbed by either the entire class or by an individual. As a result of these comparisons, standards may be established for the future. By basing measurements on these standards, teachers can readily judge the extent of student accomplishment.

It is also possible, by basing comparisons on preconceived standards, to determine the progress being made to meet course objectives. Standards are set for the knowledge required by a practicing cosmetologist. By comparing student knowledge with these standards, instructors can readily see how well their students are progressing toward becoming efficient cosmetologists. Student learning is expressed in the terms of what he (she) must know, the technical ability he must acquire and the time he needs to perform properly in the beauty salon.

PRE-TESTS USED IN PLANNING TEACHING PROGRAM

Before starting to teach a cosmetology course, it is wise to give students a pre-test. The most efficient and economical way to teach is to start your program from the point of knowledge already acquired by students. It would be a waste of time to reteach material that students already know. Much valuable time can be saved for both the teacher and student if teaching and learning begin at the proper point. The pre-test determines what students already know and then they are taught the additional subject matter they must know. The mastery tests then indicate whether or not the students have learned or acquired sufficient knowledge to advance in the course or to qualify as cosmetologists.

ESSAY QUESTIONS IN COSMETOLOGY TESTING

The traditional essay question is perhaps the most familiar type of question. However, it is the least valuable to the cosmetology teacher as an examination device.

Essay questions are the most subjective of all examining techniques and, therefore, are not recommended for use in cosmetology tests. They are a valid measurement of ability in written composition. However, the purpose of a cosmetology test is to evaluate subject matter knowledge and not writing ability.

The foremost fault of the essay examination is its lack of objectivity. The merit of the paper does not determine the grade. The examination mark is the result of the subjective judgment of the person who rates the paper at the particular moment. This has been proven time after time by numerous experiments. In one experiment, the written papers of two examinees were graded by 140 different raters. The marks ranged from 64 to 98 percent.

However, the essay question can be a valuable tool in oral questioning in the classroom. Here, instructors may ask questions which will permit students to really discuss an area of knowledge in great depth.

QUALITIES OF A GOOD EXAMINATION

A good test has the following qualities:

1. It accurately measures the student's understanding or skill.
2. The questions and directions are clear, concise and complete.
3. It is easy to give, easy to take and easy to correct.
4. Questions are valued fairly and accurately.

OBJECTIVE TYPE EXAMINATIONS IN COSMETOLOGY TRAINING

The teacher will find many advantages in using objective tests, since:

1. A great number of questions can be asked and, therefore, the entire subject matter can be quickly and adequately tested.
2. Reading and writing ability is kept at an absolute minimum so that rating is based on subject matter learned and not on the ability to write well.
3. Papers can be marked by almost anyone.
4. Marking can be done quickly.
5. Answers are either right or wrong without any guessing as to the accuracy of an answer.
6. Students are not penalized for extraneous attitudes.
7. The examination is not affected by irrelevant, outside factors.

IMPORTANT CONSIDERATIONS IN PREPARING OBJECTIVE TYPE TESTS

There are a number of different types of objective questions available to the cosmetology instructor. General characteristics which apply to every type are as follows:

1. Questions should be based on the subject matter taught.
2. Questions must be stated as clearly and briefly as possible.
3. Leading words, such as "always," "never," "all," "every" should be avoided.
4. Avoid double negatives, such as "It is **not impossible** to permanent wave tinted hair."
5. Avoid placing questions on paper so that answers appear in patterns.
6. Avoid using ambiguous questions, which in some cases may be true and, in others false.
7. Use at least four responses in multiple choice questions.
8. Eliminate ridiculous answers in multiple choice questions which permit the answering of the questions by simple deduction.
9. Avoid creating a false question by simply adding the word "not" to a positive question. It would be much wiser to prepare questions in positive manner. For example:
Infection refers to the destruction of pathogenic bacteria.   T.   F.
10. Make the examination as comprehensive as possible by asking questions in all areas of knowledge taught.
11. Test for the practical application of material learned, not only for memorized material.

EXAMINATIONS SHOULD COVER WIDE AREA

If examinations are to be valuable as part of the teaching program, sufficient time should be allocated for testing all subjects being taught. If time is devoted to teaching an item, then the instructor must take time to prove that it has been properly learned. If the subject is not tested, then there is no way of knowing whether it has been properly taught or whether the students have learned it.

WEIGHTING THE EXAMINATION

The instructor must carefully weight the examination to give greater emphasis to more important areas, and less emphasis to items of minor importance. This can be done by either giving more credit to certain questions or by using more questions on certain subjects. Students should be informed in advance if some questions carry more weight than others.

TYPES OF OBJECTIVE QUESTIONS USED IN COSMETOLOGY TESTING

In the following pages we will discuss some of the more commonly used types of objective questions employed in cosmetology teaching and testing.

1. **Completion questions**

    Completion questions are those in which a statement is presented with an important word or phrase missing. The student is required to complete the statement by supplying the word or words which will give the statement the correct meaning.

    The requirement for clean-cut brevity is one of the important merits of the completion question. It motivates the development of the ability to recall and accurately apply the subject matter learned. The exact answer required makes it possible to cover a large amount of subject matter in a relatively short period of time; thus, the sampling of cosmetology knowledge can be much greater.

    Well prepared completion questions can be less confusing, fairer because of less guessing, less likely to give the wrong impression, more thorough, and require more thought and ability than most of the other types of objective questions.

    Directions: Complete the following statements by writing the correct word in the space provided on the score sheet.

    Example: The action of the hair lightener continues as long as the hair is kept ....
    (moist)

2. **Simple recall questions**

    Simple recall questions require the use of one or more words in the answers. This type of question has all the advantages of the completion question and, in addition, does not limit you to one or two word answers. The possibilities of guessing are at a minimum because no indication of the correct answer is given in the statement. The answers must be factual and based strictly upon the student's ability to recall the correct information.

    Directions: Write the words that answer the question in the space of the score sheet opposite the item number. The number of blank lines on your test paper indicates the number of words required for the correct answer.

    Example: Hygience deals with ....
    (the preservation of health)

3. **Multiple choice questions**

    The multiple choice question is one of the most valuable of the objective type and deserves wide use. It has a number of outstanding merits. While it is more difficult to prepare, it is easy to give and to score. With the use of a key, it can be scored with great ease and rapidity. It is easy to take, definite, fair, interesting and thorough. The fact that there is less chance for guessing gives it a special appeal.

The multiple choice test consists of a series of statements with at least four responses suggested for correctly completing each. One is the correct or best response; the others are incorrect or of lesser merit. The test requires that the student recognize the correct response. This type of question demands judgment and the ability to select the best from among several possibilities.

Directions: Each of the following statements gives four responses. Select the best response and place the letter preceding it opposite the item number appearing on the score sheet.

Example: In order to determine whether or not a patron is allergic to the chemical relaxer, give a:

    a) color test   x c) patch test
    b) filler test   d) strand test

4. True-false questions

The true-false test consists of a series of statements, some of which are true and the rest are untrue. The true statements are in conformity with the facts or general principles which the student has been taught. The false statements are not in accord with the accepted facts. The test requires the student to recognize the correct and the erroneous statements and to apply this knowledge in determining which are accurate and which are not. The ability to discriminate between truth and falsity is a valid measure of the students' knowledge of the subject matter covered by the statements.

Statements must be carefully prepared so that they are definitely true or false. Any statement that can possibly be answered either way is of no value as a test item. Approximately the same number of true and false statements should be used and care must be exercised not to create a pattern of the answers.

Directions: Carefully read each statement. Some are true; others are false. If you believe that a statement is true, draw a circle around the letter T; if you believe that the statement is false, draw a circle around the letter F.

Example: A bluing rinse is used to neutralize the yellow cast in gray or white hair. .... x T   F

                After a finger wave setting, prolonged drying will result in a deeper wave. .... T   x F

5. Matching questions

Matching tests are especially important to examine the understanding of the relationships between different items. In this type of test, lists of items are arranged in opposite columns. The object of the test is to match the items in column I with the items in column II with which they are most closely associated.

Directions: Mark opposite the item number on the score sheet the letter of the item in Column II which is most closely associated with the item in Column I.

Example:

Column I	Ans.	Column II
1. baldness	d	a) keratin
2. comedone	f	b) pityriasis
3. hair	a	c) whitehead
4. dandruff	b	d) alopecia
5. canities	h	e) harden curles
		f) blackhead
		g) slithering
		h) grey hair

6. **Re-arrangement questions**

This type of question is especially valuable when testing student knowledge of the correct procedure to follow in performing a cosmetology technique.

Directions: Six steps are listed below for performing some cosmetology service. These steps are not arranged in proper order. Determine the order in which these steps should be taken and place the letter preceding it opposite the correct order number on the answer sheet.

Example: The correct procedure following in giving a patch test is:

	Answer
a) apply test solution	1. c
b) examine test area	2. f
c) wash test area	3. a
d) dry test area	4. e
e) testing period	5. b
f) allow to dry	6. d

7. **Identification questions**

Identification questions are very good for testing the ability of students to recognize and identify parts of the body or objects. This type of question is especially important in cosmetology for testing the ability to recognize the structure of various parts of the anatomy. An entire organ may be shown with parts marked. The student is required to write the names of the parts on the score sheet. These questions not only arouse interest but are very effective in testing understanding of new terms.

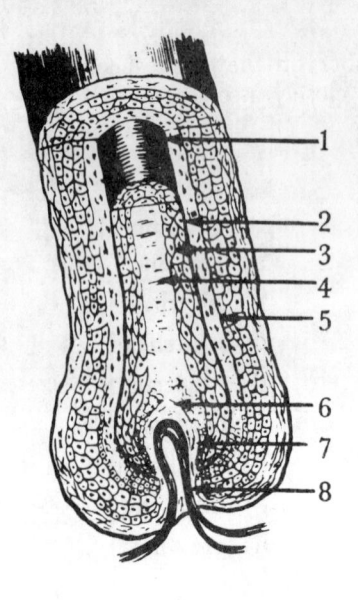

Directions: Write the names of the parts on the score sheet opposite the item numbers.

Answers
1 Hair
2 Cuticle
3 Cortex
4 Medulla
5 Hair Follicle
6 Hair Bulb
7 Hair Papilla
8 Blood Vessels

8. **Emumeration or listing questions**

This type of question can be used to great advantage by the teachers of cosmetology when they wish to test students' knowledge of lists or series of items. These questions are important because they test factual knowledge without giving any assistance to students in recognizing the answers and, therefore, call for actual knowledge of the subject.

Example: List at least four (4) implements used in hair shaping.
a) shears
b) razor
c) thinning shears
d) comb

EFFICIENT TEST OF ADMINISTRATION

Examinations should be easy to give, easy to take and easy to score. Efficiency requires that their administration be conducted as expeditiously as possible. Whenever feasible, examinations should be so organized that results can be scored in some uniform manner, as with prepared keys.

It may be accepted as somewhat axiomatic in test construction that the more time spent in the formulation of the examination, the better the quality and the greater the economy of time in scoring the test.

MEANINGFUL TESTS OF PREPARATION AND ADMINISTRATION

1. In preparing a test, the instructor must be certain that the directions given are so clear that there is not the slightest doubt as to what is required, including examples or illustrations of different types of questions. In order to maintain absolute impartiality, no one student should be given additional instructions or hints. Any oral statements should be made loud enough to be heard by all students.
2. As soon as the test has begun, the teacher should circulate throughout the room to make certain that students are following instructions. Students should be informed in advance as to whether the test is a power test, with unlimited time, or a speed test, with a definite time limit. In any event, students must know how much time will be allowed for the test.
3. Whenever possible, use identical scoring sheets for all types of tests. Scoring sheets have become so standardized that they may be applied to almost every type of question.
4. If the test is to be a true teaching device, it should be reviewed with the class after the papers are marked.
5. Students should be advised, as quickly as possible, as to the marks they have received. They should also be informed of the high, average and low marks of their group, in order that they be able to make comparisons.
6. It is inadvisable to set a passing mark before the papers are rated. The passing mark should depend upon the difficulty of the test and the results of the entire class.

INSTRUCTOR MUST DECIDE WHAT PURPOSE EXAMINATION IS TO SERVE

Each examination must have a definite purpose. If the instructor wants to find out the effectiveness of his teaching and what the class has learned, he will be unable to do so unless he can compare this with what students knew at the beginning of the course. Therefore, it is wise to give tests to discover what knowledge students have at the very beginning of the course. After the subject has been taught, another test will help to determine what they have learned. A comparison will give a true picture of the effectiveness of the teaching.

COMPARE TEST RESULTS

Test marks become significant only when they can be compared with some basic standard. Comparisons may be made with class averages or standards acceptable in trade practice. Passing or failing marks should be determined by comparison with a set basis.

EXAMINATIONS MUST BE REVISED TO MEET NEEDS—
VALIDITY OF QUESTIONS

In order that examinations be truly effective, they must be thoroughly analyzed after they have been given. If a large number of students miss certain questions, those questions must be carefully studied.

It is possible that the questions were either vague or poorly phrased. If this is discovered, they should be revised to remove all ambiguities and to improve their clarity.

This also enables the teacher to isolate those areas which have not been adequately taught. The importance of this is readily apparent because it permits the teaching method or procedure to be improved in order to insure good teaching and learning.

PERFORMANCE TESTS

A performance (practical) test is employed to decide whether or not students can perform cosmetology techniques well enough to meet the standards required by the profession. Such a test should never be just a haphazard observation of students doing certain jobs. In fact, a performance test must be carefully planned and given, if it is to provide an accurate evaluation of student accomplishments.

All practical or clinic work is a series of tests of accomplishment. Testing of cosmetology students' understanding of what to do, and how to do it, is a continuous process. In order for this type of testing to be meaningful, every effort must be exerted to make the entire process as objective as possible.

1. **Preparing the performance test.**
   a) Determine exactly which skills or techniques you wish to test.
   b) Consider safety precautions and sanitary measures.
   c) Speed.
   d) Ability to organize job.
   e) Accuracy.
   f) Exactness in performance.
   g) Manual dexterity.
   h) List a step-by-step breakdown of the entire performance.
   i) By consulting the steps or key points of the technique, decide upon the acceptable standards for each item that is to to be tested, also the relative value for each step.

j) Prepare written directions for students. These are best since they can be standardized to give each student an equal opportunity.
h) Prepare a scoring sheet. This also serves to present a standardized guide.
l) List, and make available, the supplies and equipment the students will require.

EVALUATE SKILLS BY COMPARISON

Quality of skills performed at a practical test may be evaluated and scored objectively by comparison with a set norm. In permanent waving, for example, the work performed may be compared with samples set up on mannequins. The technique can be compared with the sample and scored accordingly.

RATING THE TIME TAKEN TO COMPLETE A TASK

The element of time cannot be ignored in the marking procedure. The performance of a good quality cosmetology technique, taking only half an hour to complete, should be rated higher than another good quality performance of the same technique which takes a full hour to complete.

Time is very important in the operation of a beauty salon. The difference between making a profit and suffering a loss may be the amount of time required to perform the various services in the salon.

Time standards should be set up and marked, in addition to quality standards.

EVALUATING PERFORMANCE PROCEDURES

In teaching cosmetology, it is essential that students be taught to follow step-by-step procedures in performing the various techniques. Since following correct procedures is an objective of the course, a method of checking and testing must be employed in order to be certain that this objective is met.

PROCEDURES CHECKED BY OBSERVATION

A direct method of checking whether students follow correct procedures is by observing them while they are at work. This method enables the instructor to compare their procedures with others in the same class.

Of course, the above is a rather subjective method of rating procedures.

WRITTEN TESTS EMPLOYED TO CHECK PROCEDURES

In order to obtain more objective evaluations of the following of correct procedures by students, written examinations may be used. Employing certain type of questions will enable instructors to determine whether or not students really know the correct procedures to be followed.

The application of rearrangement or listing questions, explained earlier, provide tests of correct procedures.

Example: The correct sequence of steps to be followed in giving a patch test is

a) apply test solution   c
b) examine test area   f
c) wash test area   a
d) dry test area   e
e) testing period   b
f) allow to dry   d

True-false questions can also be used in testing for correct procedure.

Example: The last step in giving a patch test is drying the test area. (Answer: true)

The last step in giving a patch test is examining the test area. (Answer: false)

TEACHING THROUGH EVALUATION OF PROCEDURES

There are a number of reasons for the failure of students to follow the correct cosmetology procedures they have been taught.

1. The student does not know the correct procedure. This is an indication that the instruction was inadequate. In such a case it will be necessary that the student be re-taught with improved teaching techniques and special emphasis on the correct procedure to be followed.

2. The student does know the correct procedure but wants to experiment, with the hope of finding a better or easier method for performing the required skills. Under these circumstances, the student should be required to follow the procedures taught and provision made for discussion with the teacher of his or her new ideas. The student should not be denied the right to try to improve a method or procedure. Many times, teachers learn from students under these conditions.

3. The student knows the procedure taught but because he (she) has had previous experience in the practice of cosmetology is able to employ short cuts in doing the job. Under these conditions, it might be wise to review the student's situation and, perhaps, put him (her) at more advanced work.

4. The student knows the procedure taught but is thoughtless and careless, and just does not "think." Under these circumstances, the student should be admonished to use the correct procedure, and advised of the harm which might result to himself and to others, from such carelessness.

EVALUATING STUDENT PERSONALITY TRAITS

In addition to evaluating the technical skills and knowledge of students, it is important to analyze their personality traits. It may be assumed that rating clinic and classroom work will also reflect personality traits to some degree. A demonstration of initiative, self-reliance and perserverance will probably result in higher marks in practical and written examinations. However, special personality ratings will expose those students who are perfectly capable of doing good work but do not do their best because of poor attitude or other personality weaknesses. It is quite possible to compare personal qualities of students in a manner similar to comparisons of other work. Marks of personality traits should be indicated separately from those reflecting work in the classroom and in the clinic.

THE QUALITY OF TEACHING AS AFFECTED BY PERSONALITY RATINGS

1. Help instructors to better understand students.
2. Isolate weak areas in student attitudes and point out areas requiring teacher concentration.
3. Direct the application of corrective measures to relieve entire class of elements which retard progress.
4. Isolate trouble makers who detract from the overall effort of the instructor for the teaching benefit of the greater number of students.
5. Permit personal quality analysis for attention of prospective employers.

KNOWING HOW, BUT NOT APPLYING KNOWLEDGE, AN IMPORTANT ELEMENT OF FAILURE

The students who know how to perform properly but will not apply this knowledge are headed for complete failure. It isn't enough to know how to do the job properly. It is more important that students exert every effort to apply their knowledge and ability.

A very important job for the instructor is not only to teach proper cosmetology techniques but, also, to instill students with the desire and will to apply this knowledge and ability. It is the instructor's task to get students "on the beam" and rating of personality traits will assist in this very important responsibility.

THE APPLICATION OF RATING STUDENT ATTITUDES

A study of personality qualities indicates that certain characteristics are common among groups of students. These qualities may be listed and camparable ratings of groups of students developed.

The rating chart on the next page is offered as a guide to facilitate such comparisons. However, since these ratings are highly subjective, they must be handled carefully to avoid misinterpretations and misleading comparisons.

PROPER RATING OF STUDENTS

Rating: To properly rate students, add the number of points scored for each area. Then divide the total by seventy (70). This will give you the percentage rating.

Compare this rating with the following standards:

Excellent 90-100%
Good 80- 89%
Fair 70- 79%
Poor .... 69% or less

PERSONAL IMPROVEMENT PROGRAM

The sincere instructor who wishes to try to improve his students' attitudes and personalities should incorporate the subject of Personal Improvement in his program. This professional effort could result in better qualified graduates, who are more capable of effectively coping with the public.

For information on a personal improvement program for boys and girls, write to:

Milady Publishing Corp.
3839 White Plains Road
Bronx, New York 10467

RATING CHART OF STUDENT'S PERSONAL QUALIFICATIONS

Quality	SCORE 10 9 8 Excellent	SCORE 7 6 5 Good	SCORE 4 3 2 Fair to Poor
COOPERATION (Interest) (Leadership)	Always participates in collective action for common good. Observes all rules. Helps others.	Usually participates in collective action for common good. Observes most rules. Helps others when asked.	Never participates in collective action for common good. Ignores rules. Never helps others.
PROMPTNESS (Punctuality)	Always prompt in doing work. Gets to school on time. Does not quit work before time.	Generally prompt doing work. Gets to school on time most of the time. Seldom quits before time.	Usually dilatory in work. Is late most of the time. Usually quits before time.
SELF-RELIANCE (Judgment)	Relies on own efforts to solve problems. Uses discernment.	Does not call for help in problem solving most of the time.	Depends largely upon teacher for help in all work.
INDUSTRY (Drive) (Initiative) (Perseverance)	Habitually diligent. Pays steady attention to job. Steadfast and energetic.	Generally diligent. Works hard most of the time.	Takes time to loaf. Dallies about. Finds excuses for not working.
RESPONSIBILITY (Dependability)	Always gets a good job done on time. Is answerable for all assignments.	Is not always accountable to authority for work assigned.	Cannot be depended upon to do his work.
HONESTY (Reliability)	Always tell the truth. Invariably does the honorable thing.	Seldom untruthful.	Lies and cheats most of the time.
PERSONAL APPEARANCE (Boys)	Always clean, neatly dressed, clean-shaven, with clean hands and nails. Wears well-fitted and shined shoes.	Seldom unclean. Sometimes sloppy in dress, often forgets to shave.	Always dirty, usually sloppy in dress, usually unshaven.
PERSONAL APPEARANCE (Girls)	Always wears appropriate hairstyle and make-up and has smooth hands and manicured nails. Is neatly and appropriately dressed. Wears well-fitted, polished shoes and clean hose without wrinkles.	Seldom wears unsuitable hairstyle and make-up and has unclean nails and shoes. Sometimes clothes may need cleaning and do not co-ordinate.	Always wears unsuitable hairstyle and make-up, has disorderly hair and unclean hands and nails. Wears clothes in sloppy manner and shoes that are unpolished or in need of repair. Does not wear hose or if she does, they are usually wrinkled.

Personal Notations . . .

9

MAINTAINING CLASSROOM DISCIPLINE

One of the prime responsibilities of the cosmetology instructor is the maintainance of classroom discipline and deportment. For the most part, this may be only a minor problem, however, on occasion, it may become a problem of utmost importance.

The application of disciplinary measures may often be responsible for the success or failure of an instructor. The following discussion deals with the prevention of disciplinary problems and suggestions for solving them—when and if they do arise.

THE OBJECTIVE OF DISCIPLINE IS TO CORRECT

Discipline, as an educational function, is intended to correct rather than to punish. As part of the educational structure, discipline is systematic training to improve student actions and attitudes.

It is almost as important to train students in discipline as it is to train them in cosmetology skills and techniques. In addition to learning how to perform cosmetology services, students must learn how to:

1. Do the work in accordance with the supervisor's or employer's desires.
2. Be able to get along well with others, both patrons and fellow workers, while working; and
3. Carry out his (her) share of responsibilities on the job.

EMPLOY TACT AND FAIRNESS IN REPRIMANDING STUDENTS

No instructor should permit personal feelings to influence his judgment in reprimanding students. Allowing your own poor health or ill-feeling to affect your disciplinary actions may aggravate an already difficult situation. It is wise to refrain from any drastic action in the "heat of the moment." Give yourself the opportunity to cool off or to feel better before undertaking any important disciplinary action.

BE CONSISTENT IN DISCIPLINARY ACTIONS

Students should always be made to feel and understand that the same rules of discipline indiscriminately apply to all students. Instructors should never have "favorites" or "pets" who are permitted to "get away" with infractions, while others are not.

Under no circumstances should the instructor humiliate a student before others. All corrections should be made strictly impersonally and privately.

CONSIDERATION MUST BE GIVEN TO STUDENT'S MENTAL AND PHYSICAL CONDITION

Instructors know that their own physical or mental conditions often influence their actions. The same also is true of students. Therefore, teachers must be understanding and compassionate in their actions toward students.

DISCOVER REASONS FOR STUDENT'S ACTIONS

Instructors must make an effort to discover the reasons for a student's actions. Questioning may reveal that these are the result of misunderstanding, a lack of appreciation of the importance of certain activities, an absence of incentive to learn, or a real or imaginary injustice.

A STUDENT'S PAST ACTIONS SHOULD NOT INFLUENCE PRESENT TEACHER ATTITUDES

Every student must be given a fair chance to do a good job. A poor reputation, established by earlier actions, should not affect present teacher-reactions. Do not hold previous trouble over the student's head.

MEANINGFUL WORK HELPS TO MAINTAIN ORDER

A continuous supply of important work helps to maintain student interest and helps to avoid disciplinary problems. Instructors must assign meaningful tasks to challenge the ability of students. Work provided just to keep students busy soon loses its attractiveness and leads to a lessening of interest, which, in turn, helps to create classroom problems.

ARRANGE CLASS SO THAT EVERY STUDENT CAN SEE AND HEAR CLEARLY

Students will allow their interest and attention to wonder when they cannot see or hear clearly. They begin to feel that they are "left out" of the presentation. Much inattention and "horseplay" can be avoided by making certain that each student fully participates in the class program.

SUFFICIENT EQUIPMENT AND MATERIALS MUST BE PROVIDED

Students must be provided with mannequins and similar equipment and with ample supplies. If students are required to wait their turn to use essential training equipment, or if they are not kept constructively occupied at all times, their idleness may result in disciplinary problems.

INSTRUCTORS MUST STOP ANY DISORDER AS SOON AS IT STARTS

At the first sign of any disorder, the instructor must take immediate action to bring it to a halt. Arguments or "horseplay" should not be allowed since they may develop into serious situations. Any congregation or loafing of students must be broken up immediately.

MAINTAIN STRICT ATTITUDE TOWARD NEW STUDENTS

New groups of students must be handled in a strict manner. Many students "test out" a teacher to see how far they can go. If students immediately find that the teacher means business, they realize that their job is to learn and not to indulge in "horseplay." After students have been thoroughly indoctrinated with the importance of their responsibilities, teachers may become slightly more lenient.

RESPECT STUDENT'S INTERESTS AND RECOGNIZE IMPORTANCE OF THEIR PROBLEMS

Never belittle the interests or work of any student. The quickest way to discourage a student is to fail to respect his work or efforts. Encourage your students to come to you for advice and guidance.

WHENEVER POSSIBLE, HANDLE DISCIPLINARY PROBLEMS YOURSELF

It is only on very rare occasions that the good instructor is required to go to the school's administrative authorities in order to maintain discipline in his class. Discipline is the direct responsibility of the instructor and not of the school's Director or Administrator. Only those infractions which are of a very major nature should be called to the attention of the Director.

ACT AND SPEAK IN POSITIVE MANNER

As an instructor you must be sure that students perfectly understand the reasons for proceeding in certain ways. Instructions, directions or corrections should be stated in positive terms, not negatively. It is wise to say "do so and so" instead of saying "don't do so and so." If students are instructed to do a certain thing chances are that it will be done but they will do it more willingly and probably better, if the instructor carefully explains the reasons for the action. Students should be instructed to conform to regulations. It is also important that they fully understand the reasons for disciplinary action.

RULES AND REGULATIONS SHOULD BE LIMITED IN NUMBER AND STRICTLY ENFORCED

Rules should be limited in number to those that are necessary for efficient operation. They should never be made just for the sake of creating rules. Students should be fully informed as to the reason for each rule and why it must be strictly enforced.

Rules should be stated positively, whenever possible, and should not suggest wrong behavior or activities. A rule should say "All refuse must be placed in waste container," not "Do not throw refuse on the floor."

EXTRA SCHOOL WORK MUST NOT BE ASSIGNED AS PUNISHMENT

The assignment of extra, difficult work as a disciplinary weapon is contrary to the principles of good teaching and may act to destroy the interest of a student in the entire educational program. Class work, clinic work and homework should only be assigned as part of the teaching-learning pattern. These assignments should be part of a constructive program for training the professional cosmetologist and never negatively as a means of punishment.

THE ENTIRE CLASS SHOULD NOT BE PUNISHED FOR THE ACTIONS OF ONE INDIVIDUAL

An instructor could very easily create additional disciplinary problems by punishing the entire class for the actions of one individual. The resentment created by this action raises a barrier between the class and the teacher. It destroys the good teacher-student relations which may previously have been developed. The wise teacher enlists the aid of the entire class to help solve such disciplinary problems.

TEACHER-STUDENT ARGUMENTS MUST BE AVOIDED

An instructor may very easily lose the respect of the class, and thus decrease his or her teaching efficiency, by engaging in petty arguments with individual students. Students must be given the opportunity to defend themselves. However, do not enter into debates on the student's action. It is not necessary to repeat your charges against the student or to enter into long recriminations.

AVOID THE USE OF OBSCENE OR DEROGATORY LANGUAGE

The rights and pride of a student must be respected. A student should never be humiliated or angered by your abuse of him, or use of intemperate language, before his fellow-students.

It is unwise to accuse a student of being "dumb," "lazy" etc. Statements of this type do not rectify a situation and may very easily aggravate it. Better results are obtained by private discussion with a student in which he is told that he is capable of doing better work if he would exert a little more effort.

Students appreciate being called by their names. Everyone likes to be properly recognized. Student resentment may be created unnecessarily, by careless language on the part of the instructor.

Instructors should never make threats. Student respect for a teacher is quickly lowered by the fact that the teacher makes meaningless threats, which cannot be carried out. Threats, in and of themselves, act to lower teacher prestige and usually are difficult or impossible to carry out.

MAINTAIN TEACHER DIGNITY—DO NOT BECOME TOO FAMILIAR WITH STUDENTS

It is poor professional policy for the instructor to become too friendly or familiar with students. Maintaining discipline and giving instructions become increasingly difficult when the teacher becomes too friendly with students.

An instructor must create student respect by maintaining the dignity of his (her) professional status.

MAINTENANCE OF DISCIPLINE IS A COOPERATIVE EFFORT

Maintaining school discipline is the cooperative responsibility of all instructors. If students are permitted to be lax and disorderly by one teacher, it is almost impossible to have them settle down to business and act orderly for the next teacher. A good instructor does not hesitate to correct disorder either in his own class or in another when that teacher is not present.

CORRECTIVE ACTION MUST FIT THE VIOLATION COMMITTED

Great care and good judgment must be exercised by the instructor in any disciplinary action.

Students must be permitted to demonstrate that they wish to act properly and comply with school rules. Perhaps the misdeed was the result of a lack of knowledge or inexperience; all people make mistakes. It would be a great injustice to discourage a student to the point where he or she would discontinue cosmetology training because of unduly harsh penalties for relatively minor infractions.

Instructors must be especially careful to "make the punishment fit the crime."

DO NOT CREATE AN ATMOSPHERE OF FEAR

Instructors who are harsh disciplinarians may create an atmosphere which discourages students from complete participation in the educational process. It is not good teaching to subdue students to the point where they are afraid to speak their minds. Teachers must not become disciplinary tyrants, but should make every effort to find a middle road between laxity and tyranny.

INSTRUCTORS MUST NOT EMPLOY "TORTURE-CHAMBER" TACTICS

Students should not be forced into the role of informants. Teachers should not subject students to severe cross-examination in an effort to discover who was responsible for a particular action. Students do not want to inform on fellow students. Instructors should solve their disciplinary problems without resorting to espionage or "third degree" methods.

INSTRUCTORS MUST LEARN TO CONTROL THEIR TEMPERS AND NOT DISPLAY EMOTIONAL DISTURBANCES

The teacher who has temper tantrums is creating unnecessary disciplinary problems. Many times students enjoy watching the teacher's display of uncontrollable rage and excitement. It almost becomes a vaudeville act and they may deliberately create new situations which would instigate a repeat performance.

Maintain discipline but do not let students "get under your skin."

STUDENT PERSONALITY PROBLEMS

Every teacher is likely to encounter certain difficult students who require individual attention. How to handle each requires deep insight into that person's difficulty. However, the following generalizations may be helpful:

1. **The "know-it-all,"** who takes a superior attitude toward the proceedings. He may act bored and indicate that he feels his attendance is a waste of time. Students with some superficial experience in cosmetology often take this attitude at the start of the course. Often, a pre-quiz to test existing knowledge of the subject matter, or a few direct questions calling for considerable insight into a situation, will change the attitude of these students. They come to realize that there is much for them to learn.

2. **The perpetual talker,** who tries to dominate the discussion and expound upon personal experiences and knowledge. His hand is up a good deal of the time, waving for attention. From the very beginning, you the teacher must make an effort to recognize the many different types of students and not allow one student to stay in the limelight. If the "mouth" persists, it may be wise at a class "break" to talk privately with this person. Tell the student that you appreciate his interest and participation but that the others did not enroll in the school just to listen to him—that when he talks too much, it simply antagonizes the rest of the students. Point out that an occasional well-thought-out statement will get him better personal recognition.

3. **The arguer,** who is highly critical of what you say and of what others say; he is a dissenter. Such a person can be a valuable addition to any class

even though there is a tendency to try to crush him and to obtain easy, if shallow agreement. So long as he dissents on intellectual or factual lines, his points should be listened to and carefully weighed. A good plan is to draw out this student, encouraging him to tell why he believes or feels as he does. Once this student has gotten a "pet peeve off his chest," he is likely to see the point of view of others. One way to deal with such an individual is to ask members of the class to answer his arguments rather than to take issue with him yourself. Certainly, don't try to crush him with your authority, but do point out his responsibility as a member of the class group.

4. **The silent student,** "the rabbit," who has nothing to volunteer. There are many reasons for this attitude but lack of worthwhile ideas is seldom one of them. Questions should be directed to such a person and the instructor should show special respect for what he has to say. Once the individual sees that his contribution is adding to the group's thinking and interest, he is likely to continue to participate without special prompting. Even if such a student continues to maintain a passive attitude, he may be learning a great deal. Learning cannot be measured in terms of the degree of talking done by a person.

5. **The slow student.** There are some students who have difficulty in comprehending the subject matter and in keeping up with the class. You should bear in mind that for every student who admits to such difficulty there are many more who are having the same trouble. It is better to go slow, to make points doubly clear, rather than to allow the brightest student to set the pace. On the other hand, don't cater to the weakest student either. Offer to stay after class to help the individual, and encourage, rather than criticize him for "being dumb." Sometimes, it may be well to seat this person next to a smarter student who is willing to help the slow learner.

Of course, there are many other difficult types, such as the **cocksure person** who may be both a constant talker and an arguer. If given an opportunity, members of the class can often straighten out such an individual. And, there is the **disinterested student** who is there to pass away the time or to satisfy his or her parents that he or she is "in school learning a vocation." This person must be motivated in order to relate the subject matter to his own needs and interests.

10

DEVELOPING A SUBJECT TEACHING PROGRAM

A subject teaching program is a written plan or outline for directing the thinking, planning and technical training for a particular cosmetology service. A subject program is one of a number of units of study within the organized curriculum required for training the professional cosmetologist. The procedure to be followed in preparing a subject teaching program is presented in this chapter.

LIST OVERALL OBJECTIVES OF THE SCHOOL

The cosmetology instructor must be thoroughly familiar with the overall the Cosmetology State Board's curriculum and school literature should be the first step.

LIST DESIRED OBJECTIVES OF THE PARTICULAR SUBJECT

The instructor must be thoroughly knowledgeable of the broad objectives to be attained in teaching every cosmetology technique or service. These objectives must be established before embarking on the preparation of the specific program to be developed. The importance of the particular subject in the overall objectives of the course must be clearly set forth.

BECOME FAMILIAR WITH THE OBJECTIVES OF THE SPECIFIC SUBJECT

The next step in creating a subject teaching program is to list the objectives to be attained in teaching the subject. These objectives should set forth what skills the students should develop and the knowledge they must acquire. They must be specifically stated and should be reasonably attainable, considering the time, facilities and equipment available. To be worthwhile, the knowledge and skill to be developed must be practical and important in the proper training of the cosmetologist.

DETERMINE THE AMOUNT OF TIME TO BE DEVOTED

Time is a very important factor in any cosmetology training program. In allocating time to any particular subject, careful consideration must be given to the overall objectives. Questions must be resolved as to the importance of the subject in the overall picture, the scope of the subject, its importance in actual salon practice and the depth of the knowledge required.

THE STUDENT LEVEL AT WHICH THE SUBJECT IS TAUGHT

Determination must be made as to the specific point in the entire curriculum when the subject should be taught. What preliminary training must students have before starting the subject? Should it be taught to Freshman, Juniors, Seniors? What degree of cosmetology maturity should students have attained before embarking on the study of the particular subject?

DETERMINE SIZE OF CLASS FOR EFFICIENT TEACHING AND LEARNING

The effectiveness of the entire teaching program could be impaired if the class is too large. Planning should include a determination of the maximum number of students who can be handled efficiently for best results.

LIST TEACHING METHODS, EQUIPMENT AND MATERIAL TO BE USED

In order to insure the best teaching and learning procedure for the particular subject, it is wise to list in advance the teaching method to be employed, the type of equipment to be used, the materials required and the procedure to be followed.

INDICATE METHOD OF EVALUATION

Pre-determine the method to be followed in evaluating the effectiveness of the teaching and learning process. The teacher should plan to use certain tests and determine when they should be used for maximum effectiveness.

RESEARCH YOUR PROGRAM

The instructor must be completely prepared to teach the particular subject. Do some personal research for latest trends and techniques, and look through reference material for additional ideas and information.

WHENEVER POSSIBLE, USE STUDENTS TO HELP WITH PROGRAM

Plan to use some or all of your students in your program. This will arouse interest and create a cooperative learning atmosphere.

LIST TEXT PAGES AND REFERENCE BOOKS

Make a list of reference material covering the subject matter. List the chapters, pages and sections in the school textbooks and workbooks relating to it.

OUTLINE PROCEDURE TO BE FOLLOWED IN USING EQUIPMENT AND SUPPLIES

In demonstration, practice room or clinic work, outline in advance the procedure to be followed in using equipment, supplies and visual-aids for greatest effectiveness.

LIST TECHNIQUES AND SKILLS TO BE LEARNED

Plan the techniques to be taught and the cosmetology skills to be learned. List the step-by-step procedure to be followed in performing these skills or techniques.

MAKE LIST OF DRILL PROJECTS TO BE EMPLOYED IN DEVELOPING SKILL

In developing cosmetology techniques several drill sessions may be required for different parts of the program. List these drill sessions, indicating where they are to fit into the planned program and the skill each is intended to develop.

LIST THE THEORETICAL KNOWLEDGE AND RELATED INFORMATION TO BE TAUGHT

1. Theoretical information and knowledge required in order to do the job properly. Example: Structure and texture of the skin in connection with the presentation of facial massage.
2. Related information which would be helpful to your students. Example: How the action of waving lotion on the hair helps it to maintain its curled position.

PREPARE YOUR LESSON PLANS

Based on the materials contained in your subject teaching program, prepare your lesson plans for actual implementation.

KEEP TEACHING PROGRAM FLEXIBLE

It is probable that additions, subtractions and changes will have to be made in your subject teaching program after it has been in operation. The value of the program will be tested by its actual use. Any program should be kept flexible so that it may be revised as the need arises.

DEVELOPING WRITTEN INSTRUCTION SHEETS

Instruction sheets are printed aids to assist students in learning facts and properly applying this information in performing cosmetology techniques or skills. It is important to emphasize that instruction sheets are not substitutes for an instructor but serve as aids in carrying out the instructor's program. Instruction sheets become very advantageous to the teaching and learning program when they are skillfully prepared and properly used.

BASIC ADVANTAGES OF GOOD INSTRUCTION SHEETS

1. They make certain that the entire subject matter is covered. Possibilities of important omissions are materially reduced if instruction sheets are properly written and correctly used.

2. They provide uniform instructions. Teachers do not give instructions or teach a subject twice in exactly the same manner. Subtle changes, no matter how slight, could confuse and discourage students. Instruction sheets present information in exactly the same manner each time they are used.

3. They provide practice in following written instructions. In beauty salon practice, the ability to read and follow written instructions becomes very important in dealing with new products. Written instructions accompany all cosmetology products and they must be strictly followed to avoid injury to patrons.

4. They are helpful in providing for the individual differences of slow, average and fast students, and thus permit students to make progress in accordance with individual abilities.

5. They assist the instructor in handling large groups. Since students have

written instructions and are able to progress at their own rate, the instructor is free to give individual instruction where required. Opportunities for giving individuals special attention are greatly increased.

6. They help students to develop the habit of self reliance. The written sheets enable students to solve many of their own problems without continuously requiring the aid of the instructor. They help to develop the student's initiative and innate abilities.

7. They provide for the assignment of review and advance lessons without special teacher programming. Students are not required to wait for the instructor to assign new lessons. After one project or area is completed and checked by the instructor, the student is free to proceed to the next.

8. They provide students with the opportunity to review their own efforts and work without waiting for the entire class.

9. They permit the admission of students to the course at any time without fear of having missed important preliminary work.

10. They eliminate the necessity for students to ask numerous questions, since most questions may be answered by referring to the printed instruction sheets.

DISADVANTAGES OF INSTRUCTION SHEETS

The mere use of instruction sheets does not resolve all teaching problems. Unless they are designed to definitely improve upon other methods of instruction, they may present certain disadvantages.

1. The danger is present that the instructor will begin to rely too heavily upon the written instruction sheets, and may simply hand them out without comment or without the benefit of other teaching methods. A real hazard exists if the instructor continually refers all questions back to the instruction sheets. Instruction sheets are designed to assist and supplement teaching; they are not intended to replace competent instruction.

2. It is possible that students will find it difficult to understand written instructions, although they can easily follow verbal instruction.

3. The preparation and printing of instruction sheets might become too expensive to produce in the required quantities.

4. After instruction sheets are prepared, there is the tendency to avoid revisions. Thus, they may not be kept up-to-date. It is easier to revise an oral presentation than to change, rewrite and reprint instruction sheets.

5. Great care must be exercised to keep instruction sheets in their proper sequence. If by chance, they become disarranged, learning may be impaired and disjointed.

6. Instruction sheets may become detrimental if students fail to read the complete instructions and proceed with a project after reading only part of them.

7. The danger also exists that students will pay little, or no attention, to classroom instructions or demonstrations because they will depend strictly upon the instruction sheets. On the other hand, students may pay little attention to the instruction sheets and rely completely upon classroom instruction.

MAKE INDUSTRY SURVEY FOR EXISTING INSTRUCTION SHEETS

Before proceeding to write new instruction sheets, it is wise to make a search for existing printed sheets which may contain exactly what you need. A great deal of time and money may be saved by taking advantage of instruction sheets which have already been prepared.

A good source for modern Cosmetology Instruction Sheets is the:

Milady Publishing Corp.
3839 White Plains Road
Bronx, New York 10467

TYPES OF INSTRUCTION SHEETS

There are several types of instruction sheets which can be of great benefit to cosmetology instructors. The ones mostly used in cosmetology training are:

1. Procedure sheets, which set forth the step-by-step procedure to be followed in performing cosmetology techniques.

2. Practice sheets, which set forth definite tasks for students' performance and practice drill.

WRITING PROCEDURE SHEETS

The procedure sheet sets forth the step-by-step instructions for performing a manipulative technique. It also contains the related information required for the actual performance of the technique. Each operation involved should be represented by a special procedure sheet.

1. Select a specific title of the topic. The title should describe the operation. For example: "Preparing for a Creme Rinse" or "Setting Up a Manicure Table." These titles are descriptive and state the exact tasks covered.

2. Make a list of the implements and supplies required for the performance of this task.

3. List the steps of performance in their proper sequence.

4. List the safety measures and precautions necessary to avoid injury to the patron or damage to her clothes.

5. List of test items could be compiled or source where they can be located in the Textbook, Workbook or Exam Review booklet.

MATERIAL COMPOSITION OF INSTRUCTION SHEETS

If any instruction sheets are to be used over and over again, or handled constantly by instructors or students and then returned for future use, they should be made of durable material, capable of withstanding such constant handling.

However, if the instruction sheets are to be distributed to students to become part of their notes and records, they should be prepared on ordinary paper.

The master instruction sheets, from which all duplications are made, should always be prepared on durable material.

FILING OF INSTRUCTION SHEETS

All types of instruction sheets must be readily accessible to both instructors and students. The system developed for their safe keeping must be one which also provides for easy accessibility. Instructors must be able to locate desired sheets without time-wasting searches. An index system should be used which is clearly visible and easy to maintain. Instruction sheets should be easy to obtain and easy to replace.

FLEXIBILITY OF INSTRUCTION SHEETS

Any type of instruction sheet is valuable only if it is clearly understood and technically correct. Changes in teaching methods or cosmetology techniques require that periodic revisions be made in instructional material. It may become necessary to revise certain sections to clarify statements or to bring material up-to-date. Unless such required changes are made, the instruction sheets soon become antiquated and lose much of their value.

CONCLUSION

There is no easy, guaranteed road to becoming a successful cosmetology teacher. The mere fact that an instructor reads this text does not insure his or her acquiring great instructional ability. The reading of this text will not automatically create a qualified instructor. However, success as an instructor is dependent upon the application of the concepts, precepts and techniques set forth herein.

Instructors are urged to consider carefully the principles presented, to think seriously about them and to discuss them thoroughly with fellow instructors. Of far greater importance, apply these principles to the daily work of teaching. To a great degree, success as an instructor will be measured by the extent of this application.

Personal Notations . . .